Medi-Cross II

50 Advanced Medical Terminology Crossword Puzzles

for Medical, Pre-Med, Nursing, Chiropractic, EMTs, PTs and Other Health Care Professionals and Crossword Lovers

John McLeod

Introduction

Medi-Cross II is a continuation of Medi-Cross: 100 Medical Terminology Crossword Puzzles. It is another challenging book of crosswords focused in the areas of anatomy, physiology, biology and all sciences relating to the human body.

The formation of medical terms, usually of Latin and Greek origin, enabled scientists to accurately describe the structures, functions and conditions of the body by combining word roots, prefixes and suffixes.

Medi-Cross puzzle books were created to assist in the learning and understanding of how medical terms were developed and why they are used, in a fun, non-textbook format that can be taken anywhere for study or review.

Linguistic and etymology enthusiasts will find these puzzles interesting and informative, as will students and practitioners of the health sciences.

1

1	2	3	4	■	5	6	7	8	9	■	10	11	12	13
14				■	15					■	16			
17				■	18					■	19			
20				21						22				
■	■	■	23					■	■	24				
25	26	27				■	■	28	29			■	■	■
30				■	■	31	32				■	33	34	35
36				37	38						39			
40			■	41					■	■	42			
■	■	■	43				■	■	44	45				
46	47	48			■	■	49	50				■	■	■
51					52	53						54	55	56
57				■	58					■	59			
60				■	61					■	62			
63				■	64					■	65			

Across

1. ____tive; purgative
5. Covered with hair
10. ____genesis; sexual reproduction
14. ____tia; denoting lack of force
15. Kidney waste product
16. ____olic; growth enhancing steroid
17. ____ated; charged with iron
18. Joint type at atlas and axis
19. Narrow elevation of a bone
20. Study of ecologic influences on human health
23. Prefix meaning 'green'
24. Skeleton parts
25. Inflammation of the ear
28. Spleen
30. ____phobia; fear of fatigue or overworking
31. Anterior legs
33. Blood flow imaging technique (abbrev.)
36. Within the epithelial cells
40. ___osis; production of gas in the tissues
41. A rinsing or cleansing
42. Seaweed
43. ____itis; inflammation in the womb
44. Instrument for tamponing
46. Perceive flavour in the mouth
49. _____coid; wormlike
51. Between the metacarpal bones
57. ____rhea; liquid feces
58. _____emia; lack of blood leukocytes
59. ____phobia; fear of certain places
60. ____latory; able to walk about
61. Faculty of perceiving a stimulus
62. Relating to urine
63. ____itude; a sense of weariness
64. Group of eight
65. Suffering from disease

Down

1. Quality that distinguishes a vital body from a dead body
2. ____dotal; based on case histories
3. ___derma; dryness of the skin
4. That which raises
5. Central, black, iris orifices
6. _____malacia; softening of the iris
7. Detoxifying organ
8. ____aly; deviation from normal
9. ____form; resembling a network
10. Four quarts
11. Negatively charged ion
12. Skin disease of domestic animals
13. Follows orders
21. 21st letter of the Greek alphabet
22. Excessively overweight
25. Suffix referring to 'having a condition of'
26. A sound of distinct frequency
27. ____insic; of internal origin
28. ____iasis; formation of gall or kidney stones
29. Isonicotinic acid hydrazide (abbrev.)
31. Spiked projection from a bone
32. Not hers
33. Mammary gland secretion
34. Violent anger
35. Like a wing
37. _____birth; birth material expelled
38. ___ment; constituent part
39. A bundle or fascicle of muscular fibres
43. Womb
44. Pouchlike cavity
45. Wing-like process
46. Alternately rising and falling
47. The soul or life
48. Pierces with a pointed instrument
49. A mold for keeping a skin graft in place
50. A reason for a condition
52. ____chism; a taste for suffering
53. ____tive; not essential
54. Openings or foramina
55. ____otomy; incision into an apical structure
56. A curl of hair

Across

1. Emits a low, continuous murmur
5. ___nition; elements of perception
8. A group of eight
13. Enterotoxigenic Escherichia coli (abbrev.)
14. Tender
15. _____humeral; shoulder joint
16. Food consumed at regular intervals
17. ____uria; extravasation of urine
18. Internal layer of protective material
19. Involving both the arterioles and the veins
22. Disease-spreading rodents
23. International sensitivity index (abbrev.)
24. Negatively charged ions
27. Isoelectric point (abbrev.)
29. Abbreviation for chicken embryo lethal orphan (virus)
33. not fluid
34. _____pyesis; suppuration in bone
36. ___brain; mesencephalon
37. Incision of the sclera and iris
40. U.S. doctors gp.
41. dura _____; outer brain and spinal cord membrane
42. _____itis; inflammation of the optomeninx
43. Specific sites
45. Small collapsible bed
46. ______gastria; absence of a stomach opening
47. Auditory brainstem response (abbrev.)
49. ____nestic; assisting the memory
50. Inflammation of the stomach and intestines
58. _____phobia; fear of public places
59. Injure
60. ____ambulic; pertaining to sleepwalking
61. Referring to a charged particle
62. ____tropic; directed against the cause
63. Dull, steady pain
64. _____oid; pulley-shaped
65. Cathode ray oscilloscope (abbrev.)
66. Complete bend in a vessel forming a circular ring

Down

1. ____chrome; the coloring matter of the blood
2. ____itis; inflammation in the womb
3. ____itis; inflammation of an opening
4. Of scarlike texture
5. ____trum; initial breast fluid
6. Spoken
7. ____blast; nucleus of the fertilized oocyte
8. Eyes provocatively
9. Treatment facility
10. ____dynia; sinew pain
11. ____rysm; blood vessel dilation
12. ____algia; pain in the back
14. Expectorates
20. Governed by chance
21. A venomous snake
24. _____ism; absence of saliva
25. _____cyte; healthy red blood cell
26. _____ crest; pelvic ridge
27. A small cluster of cells
28. ____nal; everlasting
30. To give expression to feeling
31. A boundary or end
32. _____meter; pain measuring instrument
34. Prefix meaning 'eight'
35. Vessel in which substances are ground with a pestle
38. ____iliac; posterior, pelvic joint
39. Final
44. Pertaining to medicine
46. _____phobia; fear of the wind
48. _____ium; arm
49. _____megaly; enlargement of an atrium
50. Manner of walking
51. ____aphobia; fear of public places
52. ____motor; related to movements caused by sound
53. Enterohemorrhagic Escherichia coli (abbrev.)
54. ____emia; presence of sodium in the blood
55. ____phobia; fear of childbirth
56. ____roid; denoting a thin purulent discharge
57. Walking unit

1	2	3	4	■	5	6	7	8	9	■	10	11	12	13
14				■	15					■	16			
17				■	18					■	19			
20				21						22				
■	■	■	23					■	■	24				
25	26	27				■	■	28	29			■	■	■
30				■	■	31	32				■	33	34	35
36				37	38						39			
40			■	41					■	■	42			
■	■	■	43				■	■	44	45				
46	47	48			■	■	49	50				■	■	■
51					52	53						54	55	56
57				■	58					■	59			
60				■	61					■	62			
63				■	64					■	65			

Across

1. Nerve branches

5. In utero development after the eighth week

10. ____dynia; labor pains

14. Prefix meaning 'name'

15. _____virus; disease transmitted by rodents

16. ____olic; growth enhancing steroid

17. ____ianism; sapphism

18. Stupid person

19. Narrow elevation of a bone

20. Study of ecologic influences on human health

23. Walking sticks

24. Skeleton parts

25. Norepine______; a neurotransmitter

28. ____rant; deviating

30. Restore to health

31. tablets

33. Adenosine 5-diphosphate (abbrev.)

36. Involving both the arterioles and the veins

40. Abbreviation for Chief of Staff

41. Medial forearm bones

42. ____gate; to wash out

43. ____genesis; development of life from nonlife

44. Pertaining to the distal portion of the large intestine

46. _____phobia; fear of one's own voice

49. _____biology; study of germ-free animals

51. Condition in which a parasite develops within a previously existing parasite

57. ____ture; an opening

58. Acronym for as low as reasonably achievable

59. ____phobia; fear of different mental conceptions

60. ____enital; present at birth

61. Light beam device

62. ____sightedness; myopia

63. Suffix meaning 'examination'

64. Suffix meaning 'seizure'

65. Consumes

Down

1. Behavior pattern individuals present to others

2. ____dotal; based on case histories

3. ____philia; pathological interest in filth

4. A mentally deficient person

5. An extreme scarcity of food

6. To wear away

7. _____ major; arm adductor

8. ____aly; deviation from normal

9. ____ary; adapted for tearing

10. Paleness

11. Negatively charged ion

12. The difference between the limits of a variable

13. Follows orders

21. ___phobia; fear of everything

22. Excessively overweight

25. ____oid; lens-shaped

26. A man distinguished by exceptional courage

27. Disease-spreading rodents

28. Plant derived juice used on skin

29. Abbreviation for bovine leukemia virus

31. ____phobia; fear of fatigue or overworking

32. Abbreviation for insulin-like activity

33. ____algia; main artery pain

34. Prefix meaning 'hard'

35. ____osis; falling out of the hair

37. Redness

38. ___acus; hip flexor

39. Poisonous volatile alkaloid derived from tobacco

43. State of immune unresponsiveness

44. A beadlike structure

45. ___ology; study of disease causes

46. _____malacia; softening of the lens

47. _____epsia; impaired digestion

48. Unobstructs

49. Take securely and hold firmly

50. Nostrils

52. ____esthesia; perception of vibration

53. Winglike structures

54. A mental conception

55. A sitting surface

56. Death

1	2	3	4	5	■	6	7	8	■	9	10	11	12	13
14					■	15			■	16				
17					■	18			19					
20					■	21						■	■	■
■	■	22			■	23				■	24	25	26	27
28	29			■	30				■	■	31			
32			■	33				■	34	35				
36			37				■	38						
39						■	40				■	41		
42				■	■	43				■	44			
45				■	46				■	47			■	■
■	■	■	48	49					■	50			51	52
53	54	55							■	56				
57					■	58			■	59				
60					■	61			■	62				

Across

1. _____ation; irregular skin tear
6. Electromyogram (abbrev.)
9. Small, egglike structures
14. Acronym for as low as reasonably achievable
15. Abbreviation for fever of unknown origin
16. Derived from wine
17. _____tosis; prolapse of the large intestine
18. Speech sound made by forcing the air stream through a narrow orifice
20. _____form; roof-shaped
21. Emergency Medical Treatment and Labor Act (abbrev.)
22. Assitance
23. Acronym for compartment of uncoupling of receptor and ligand
24. ____itis; inflammation of an opening
28. ____ular; sphincteral muscle shape
30. ____phia; a wasting away
31. ____grity; soundness of structure
32. ___lingus; sexual stimulation of the anus
33. ____taxis; slight hemorrhage
34. Musculoskeletal connective tissue
36. A convulsive or involuntary tremor
38. Individuals
39. Cerumen
40. Prefix referring to the basin-shaped hip structure
41. ___pragia; diminished functional activity in a part
42. ____cus; hip flexor
43. ____melia; congenital deformity of the limbs
44. Lacrimal gland secretion
45. ____sightedness; myopia
46. ____osis; swelling of the eye lining
47. ___iculation; joint
48. Girl
50. _____lepsy; excessive sleep disorder
53. Pain affecting one entire half of the body
56. Negatively charged ion
57. To have life
58. ___egumentary, relating to the skin
59. A stairlike structure
60. Concave parts of the hands
61. Mature
62. _____cephalon; endbrain

Down

1. ____ose; milk sugar
2. Plant derived juice used on skin
3. Calcium salts in urine
4. Lustful
5. Fast
6. Organ that responds to a nerve impulse
7. Abnormal heart sounds
8. ______genic; causing goiter
9. Egg-shaped
10. Organic substances that are essential nutrients
11. Prefix meaning 'one'
12. Roman 54
13. Angiotensin-converting enzyme (abbrev.)
19. Unit of food energy (abbrev.)
25. Referring to the uterine lining
26. Lack of muscle tone
27. ______ fascia latae; thigh abductor
28. Main protein found in milk
29. Inspire
30. Tip of a structure
33. U.S. dental grp.
34. ____phase; final stage of mitosis or meiosis
35. Expiratory reserve volume (abbrev.)
37. The condition of stunted growth
38. To pass through a membrane
40. A stripping off of epidermis
43. Eating (suffix)
44. Sleeplike state of altered consciousness
46. Cell-mediated lymphocytotoxicity (abbrev.)
47. _____omosis; blood vessel coalescence
49. Consumes
51. ____otomy; cutting operation in the vagina
52. ____ism; coitus interruptus
53. ___atitis; liver inflammation
54. ___cerbation; increased severity of a disease
55. ___phosis; loss of the eyelashes

Across

1. _____malacia; softening of the lens
6. ____algia; gland pain
10. A tubular passage
14. _____apnia; decreased arterial carbon dioxide tension
15. _____philia; a liking for fats
16. _____tive; purgative
17. Relating to a toothache
19. _____ectomy; surgical removal of part of the iris
20. Perceives flavour in the mouth
21. ___acus; hip flexor
22. _____form; resembling bone
23. An eggshell
25. _____phobia; fear of darkness
26. Fluorescence in situ hybridization (abbrev.)
30. _______genic; causing asthma
32. Relating to the intestine
35. Ocellus
39. Hard, white tooth covering
40. Prefix meaning 'farther from the midline'
41. Relating to an automaton
43. Hair and nail scleroprotein
44. Injury
46. Treat an anatomic structure with a light beam device
47. ______phobia; fear of small skin parasites
50. ______itis; penis head inflammation
53. Prefix meaning 'one billionth'
54. ___itis; inflammation of gastric cellular tissue
55. A sharp, puncturing instrument
60. Anionic neutrophil-activating peptide (abbrev.)
61. Tendency of two bodies to approach each other
63. _____atry; study and treatment of speech disorders
64. The cheek
65. Respond to a stimulus
66. _____emia; presence of sugar in blood
67. Lost blood
68. ______diagnosis; serum diagnosis

Down

1. ____esthesis; light sensitivity
2. ____toid; resembling water
3. ____taxis; slight hemorrhage
4. ____agious; communicable
5. Group of eight
6. Acute lymphocytic leukemia (abbrev.)
7. Fingers or toes
8. To remove hair
9. ____ceptor; free nerve ending that detects pain
10. Relating to the ilium and ribs
11. Prefix referring to the ankle
12. To have life
13. Transmitter or receiver
18. Suffix meaning 'enzyme'
24. A pouch
25. A thin specimen for examination
26. ____ disease; acrodynia
27. ____cent; free from wrong
28. Pierce with a pointed instrument
29. Relating to the mechanism by which blood cells attract phagocytic cells
31. ____phobia; fear of forests
33. ______grade; moving backward
34. ____cus; hip flexor
36. Prefix signifying one quadrillion
37. Fetor ____; halitosis
38. A sound of distinct frequency
42. Pertaining to the elbow
43. ___emia; presence of potassium in the blood
45. A covering layer
47. _____esia; pain insensibility
48. A narrow passage
49. _____sis; scientific investigation
51. ___biosis; resuscitation
52. _____phobia; fear of dying
54. ____dacism; disarticulation of the letter L
56. ____nal; everlasting
57. ____rhea; liquid feces
58. ____iorrhea; excessive, post-childbirth, vaginal discharge
59. ____blast; a cell nucleolus
62. Unit of energy absorbed from ionizing radiation

Across

1. _____genesis; milk production
6. Walking stick
10. Terminal portion of the upper limb
14. _____al; situated near the kidney
15. ____rysm; blood vessel dilation
16. ____esis; involuntary discharge of urine
17. _____praxia; failure of nerve conduction without structural change
18. Mark left after healing
19. ____xeny; change of host by a parasite
20. Injurious to health
22. International Commission on Radiological Protection (abbrev.)
23. International normalized ratio (abbrev.)
24. The testis
26. Sudden burst of light or heat
29. The liver
31. The broad, flaring portion of the hip bone
32. Holds back in uncertainty
36. ____atomic; denoting five atoms per molecule
37. Severe abdominal pain causing crying
38. Anything that exerts a harmful influence
39. Surgical destruction of the 10th cranial nerve
41. Smallest image-forming unit of a video display
42. Material which gloves and condoms are made from
43. Cranial cavity mass
44. ______dynia; pain in the spleen
47. ___dynia; earache
48. Infusions or decoctions
49. A muscle that produces wrinkles
56. Hooked anatomical processes
57. A tubular passage
58. Anal injection of fluid
59. ____chondria; energy producing organelles
60. Diffuse idiopathic skeletal hyperostosis (abbrev.)
61. Live-in child-care worker
62. Ache
63. ____genous; originating outside the organism
64. _____iform; Y-shaped, U-shaped

Down

1. ____ary; adapted for tearing
2. ____algia; gland pain
3. Leglike part
4. Prefix signifying one trillion
5. Coitus interruptus
6. ______ation; gonad removal
7. Antineutrophil cytoplasmic antibodies (abbrev.)
8. ____sightedness; myopia
9. Wide-eyed
10. Unilateral headache
11. _____oic; echo-free
12. _____tive; capable of nourishing
13. Medicine doses
21. Isonicotinic acid hydrazide (abbrev.)
25. Disease-spreading rodent
26. Hair insect
27. ____ually; toward the tongue
28. A self-inflicted injury
29. Spiral in form
30. Suffix meaning 'condition'
31. Inactivated poliovirus vaccine (abbrev.)
32. A section of open-ended, flexible tubing
33. ____phobia; fear of being poisoned
34. ____cephaly; cranium defect with the brain exposed
35. ___uresis; urinary excretion of sodium
37. An agent destructive to cells
40. ___ugo; fine fetal body hair
41. An offspring or descendant
43. British thermal unit (abbrev.)
44. Extremity of a limb left after amputation
45. _____phobia; fear of poverty
46. _____ferous; yielding milk
47. _____diagnosis; serum diagnosis
50. Aural
51. Repose after exertion
52. Anionic neutrophil-activating peptide (abbrev.)
53. Method of reducing pain by electric current (abbrev.)
54. Prefix meaning 'universally'
55. Unit of acoustic impedance

Across

1. Abbreviation for acetaminophen
5. ____emia; intestinal autointoxication
9. ____pedic; clubfooted
13. Prefix meaning 'one billionth'
14. Minute openings of the skin
16. Enteroinvasive Escherichia coli (abbrev.)
17. Female breasts (slang)
18. A group of plants living in the water
19. Consciousness that originates in the brain
20. _____derma; looseness and atrophy of the skin
22. Indigestion
24. ____iform; wedge-shaped
26. _____grade; moving backward
27. Target response
30. Pertaining to the distal spine
33. Pertaining to the female external genitalia
35. _____dontia; presence of supernumerary teeth
37. His bundle electrogram (abbrev.)
38. A delimited area
41. Suffix meaning 'condition' or 'state'
42. Referring to the kidney
45. Excessive calcium in the blood
48. Internal environment stimulus creating imbalance
51. To press down
52. _____oid; resembling jaundice
54. ____ivore; flesh eating mammal
55. Showing feelings
59. _____genic; causing disease
62. The soft inner substance of a hair
63. Lesser
65. Cauda
66. Smallest unit of an element
67. Suffix meaning 'pain'
68. ____versible; permanent
69. ____melia; congenital deformity of the limbs
70. Abbreviation for eye, ear, nose, and throat
71. ____lysis; the destruction of cells

Down

1. ____gonist; agonist's opposer
2. Ache
3. A precursor
4. The position of the body
5. Health resort
6. Having a uncomfortably lower than normal temperature
7. _____ia; silver poisoning
8. Tantalizes
9. _______mandibular joint; jaw jointt
10. Sup. rectus femoris attachment pt.
11. ____tive; a demulcent remedy
12. International Classification of Diseases (abbrev.)
15. Sagittal partitions dividing the nasal airways
21. ____ism; coitus interruptus
23. Endoscopic retrograde cholangiopancreatography (abbrev.)
25. Concludes
27. ____itis; eyebrow region dermatitis
28. Region surrounding the external genitalia
29. To elicit a tendon reflex
31. Nutritive
32. The subsiding of acute disease symptoms
34. Any whitish, milklike liquid
36. Tumors (suffix)
39. Abbreviation for coronary artery disease
40. ____tive; not essential
43. _______mania; morbid impulse to count
44. ____thin; emulsifying phospholipid
46. Continuous positive airway pressure (abbrev.)
47. Having no fixed or regular course
49. A mouthlike opening
50. Characteristic of old age
53. The difference between the limits of a variable
55. Abbreviation for expiratory positive airway pressure
56. Insect parasite that causes scabies
57. Pertaining to the ear
58. Lumbus
60. ____ellous; resembling fine hairs
61. Prefix meaning 'oil'
64. Disease-spreading rodent

8

Across

1. ____cine; science of healing

5. Detoxifying organ

10. ____olic; growth enhancing steroid

14. Protein synthesis coding region of DNA

15. Kidney waste product

16. ____men; earwax

17. ____osis; state of stupor

18. Overcomes difficulties

19. ____algia; homesickness

20. Abnormally large concentration of blood insulin

23. Devoid of anything extraneous

24. To look fixedly

25. A skin eruption

26. ___dontia; absence of teeth

27. Abbreviation for crown-heel (length) of fetus

28. ___otomy; surgical division of cranial nerve X

31. A device for accomplishing an end

33. ______phobia; fear of pointed objects

36. To fill or stuff

37. Relating to the intestines and kidneys

40. ____iform; weblike

42. A diaphragmatic spasm

43. ______osis; absence of sweat glands

46. ___axial; having all the axes alike

47. Computed tomography angiography (abbrev.)

50. Clinical Laboratory Assistant (abbrev.)

51. Anti____; poison-stopping substance

54. _____itis; penis head inflammation

56. ___algia; ankle pain

57. Instrument for performing mediate auscultation

60. Relating to urine

62. ______oma; artery wall mass

63. ____aly; deviation from normal

64. ____genic; idiopathic

65. Give medical aid to

66. ____form; resembling a network

67. Lower limbs between the knees and the ankles

68. Soil

69. A mental conception

Down

1. ______ocyte; sickle cell

2. ______esis; an eruption or rash

3. Toward the back

4. _____vation; a bending inward

5. ____fugal; avoiding light

6. Fe

7. A venomous snake

8. Anal injection of fluid

9. Stand firm against

10. ___emia; congenital absence of legs

11. Newborn

12. Toxic metal found in some Chinese and Ayurvedic herbal remedies

13. Gluteal

21. _____ation; support on a cushion of air

22. U.S. hospital gp.

29. Angiotensin-converting enzyme (abbrev.)

30. Growth hormone releasing hormone (abbrev.)

32. Continuous positive airway pressure (abbrev.)

33. Prefix meaning 'against'

34. ___ety; any equal part

35. ____itis; inflammation of the testis

37. Breathing out

38. Prefix meaning 'habitat'

39. Diminishes sensation

40. Caused by touch

41. Increase in size

44. Dental Surgion (abbrev.)

45. Turn around an axis

47. Copied

48. ______ment; percussive massage movement

49. Decrease in red blood cells

52. Prefix meaning 'four'

53. Used as an early anaesthetic

55. _____cide; mite-destroying agent

58. Warmth

59. ____uria; normal urination

61. Abbreviation for Chief of Staff

9

Across

1. Round, flat anatomical structure
5. ____itis; blood vessel inflammation
9. _____ectopia; floating spleen
14. ____algesia; pain caused by the merest touch
15. Sperm
16. _____metra; gas in the uterine cavity
17. ____esis; involuntary discharge of urine
18. Unadulterated
19. The dissolution or destruction of cells
20. Inflammation of the skin of the extremities
23. ____genesis; reproduction by segmentation
24. Prefix meaning 'habitat'
25. Covering layers
28. ____atry; study and treatment of speech disorders
30. Insane
33. ____itis; inflammation of an opening
34. _____tum; tooth root cover
35. ___mia; decrease in red blood cells
36. Inflammation of the fallopian tube lining
40. Roman fifty-two
41. _____osis; failure of ossification
42. Prefix meaning 'half'
43. ___ation; bowel movement
44. ____loid; cup-shaped
45. ______algia; chest pain
47. Abbreviation for electrocerebral silence
48. ____algia; proctalgia
49. Serum diagnosis
56. The legs
57. High osmolar contrast medium (abbrev.)
58. ____mania; hypochondriacism
59. Lesser
60. ____roma; artery wall mass
61. Fe
62. _____cyte; star-shaped cell
63. Ache
64. ____bellum; movement coordinator

Down

1. Abbreviation for dehydroepiandrosterone
2. Abbreviation for International Anatomical Nomenclature Committee
3. A spiked projection from a bone
4. ________genous; producing colour
5. Rough
6. _____dynia; nerve pain
7. A pathogenic microorganism
8. A mental conception
9. Attachment of one DNA molecule to another
10. _____medicine; herbal medicine
11. Dissolution (prefix)
12. Suffix meaning 'condition'
13. ___ophobia; fear of disease
21. Abbreviation for diethyltryptamine
22. _____cephalon; endbrain
25. To perceive an odor
26. Any anatomic bandlike structure
27. A point of origin
28. Suffix meaning 'seizure'
29. ____osis; direct nuclear division
30. Dura _____; outer brain and spinal cord membrane
31. The soul or life
32. _____cated; dried out
34. End result of coagulation
37. ________lytic; capable of breaking down sugar
38. _____gnosia; denial of a neurological deficit
39. Having equal tension
45. A covering structure or roof
46. Hydrocyanic acid (abbrev.)
47. A defect in structure or function
48. _____centesis; lumbar puncture
49. Fetor ____; halitosis
50. The smallest of a litter
51. Abbreviation for dihydroxyacetone phosphate
52. 9th letter in the Greek alphabet
53. Tender
54. ____rhea; maintenance of water equilibrium
55. A unit of perceived loudness
56. Abbreviation for Certified Medical Assistant

1	2	3	4	5	■	6	7	8	9	■	10	11	12	13
14					■	15				■	16			
17					18					19				
20								■	■	21				
■	■	■	22			■	■	23	24			■	■	■
25	26	27		■	28	29	30					31	32	33
34				■	■	35					■	36		
37			■	■	38					■	■	39		
40			■	41					■	■	42			
43			44						45	■	46			
■	■	■	47				■	■	48	49		■	■	■
50	51	52			■	■	53	54				55	56	57
58					59	60								
61				■	62				■	63				
64				■	65				■	66				

Across

1. Dull pains
6. 10th cranial nerves
10. ____rated; torn
14. _____genetic; producing bile
15. Abbreviation for expiratory positive airway pressure
16. ____emia; absence of oxygen in arterial blood
17. A malignant neoplasm arising from vascular endothelial cells
20. Feelings
21. Characteristic of mankind
22. Abbreviation for islet cell antibody
23. Anterior border of tibia
25. An anular flare of light surrounding a luminous body
28. Prepared with or containing milk sugar
34. ____ine; an amino acid
35. The trunk
36. Angiotensin-converting enzyme (abbrev.)
37. Automatic gain control (abbrev.)
38. _____oid; resembling water
39. Abbreviation for Brinell hardness number
40. Decay
41. A bodily distribution area
42. A long, narrow opening
43. 5th cranial nerve
46. ____dynia; sinew pain
47. Part of a surface
48. Abbreviation for international sensitivity index.
50. Opening where blood vessels and nerves enter organs
53. Nares
58. Subnormal concentration of spermatozoa in the semen
61. The insect parasite that causes scabies
62. Concludes
63. Central, black orifice in the iris
64. Infection-associated hemophagocytic syndrome (abbrev.)
65. Angiotensin-converting enzyme inhibitors (abbrev.)
66. Bifurcated

Down

1. Dull, steady pain
2. ____osis; swelling of the eye lining
3. ____tonic; of uniform tension
4. State of euphoria
5. Pertaining to sound
6. A return blood vessel
7. ____taxis; slight hemorrhage
8. Flatulence
9. Abbreviation for isopropyl alcohol
10. A small, hollow space
11. ____aly; deviation from normal
12. Brain state of total unresponsiveness to all external stimuli
13. ____thropic; originating outside the human body
18. An objective an organism seeks to attain
19. _____dynia; nose pain
23. Covering layers
24. ____ology; study of the structure of tissues
25. Highly active antiretroviral therapy (abbrev.)
26. _____ mortis; cooling of a body after death
27. _____ferous; yielding milk
29. Deviation from the normal
30. Triplet
31. An arrangement of data in parallel columns
32. Prefix meaning 'spiny'
33. _____alveolitis; periodontal disease
38. ____ralopia; day blindness
41. _____pathy; any skin disorder
42. Apparatus on which to rest the foot
44. Measures
45. To mispronounce the sibilants S and Z
49. Walking units
50. ____cide; the killing of another human being
51. ____cus; hip flexor
52. ____iasis; formation of gall or kidney stones
53. A small round structure
54. ____form; resembling bone
55. ____osion; a bursting inward
56. Roman fifty-three
57. Sodium chloride
59. Cornsilk
60. ___ology; study of tumors

1	2	3	4	■	5	6	7	8	9	■	10	11	12	13
14				■	15					■	16			
17				■	18					■	19			
20				21						22				
■	■	■	23					■	■	24				
25	26	27				■	■	28	29			■	■	■
30				■	■	31	32				■	33	34	35
36				37	38						39			
40			■	41					■	■	42			
■	■	■	43				■	■	44	45				
46	47	48			■	■	49	50				■	■	■
51					52	53						54	55	56
57				■	58					■	59			
60				■	61					■	62			
63				■	64					■	65			

Across

1. Lateral attachment of inguinal ligament (abbrev.)
5. co_____ion; sexual intercourse
10. Skin eruption
14. _____aneus; heel bone
15. _____virus; disease transmitted by rodents
16. _____blast; a cell nucleolus
17. Suffix referring to 'having a condition of'
18. _____tomy; removal of fatty tissue
19. Shape
20. Inability to feel writing on the skin
23. _____ergic; having different effects
24. Outer
25. Having many projections or protuberances
28. _____ilage; joint covering
30. _____roid; resembling a dream
31. Express grief or sorrow
33. Cradle ___; infant scalp disease
36. Intestinal organism (2 words)
40. ___egumentary; relating to the skin
41. Inter_____ dorsales; hand muscles
42. _____form; resembling bone
43. A small biting fly
44. Pertaining to a rib
46. Cisterna _____; thoracic duct origin
49. Sudden, involuntary muscle contraction
51. ____________emia; low blood cholesterol
57. Expanded disability status scale (abbrev.)
58. Relating to sheep
59. _____phobia; fear of certain places
60. Rainbow-like eye part
61. _____stry; study of teeth
62. _____pexy; surgical fixation of ileum
63. _____chezia; emotional discharge gained by uttering indecent words
64. Body structure with a specific function
65. Acronym for centromeric protein

Down

1. U.S. OB/GYN gp.
2. _____ophagous; feeding on decaying matter
3. _____cus; hip flexor
4. Boat-shaped wrist bone
5. Roof of the mouth
6. Kidney waste product
7. A person with Hansen disease
8. _____thesia; lack of sensation
9. Sensitive aesthetic perception
10. Restore to the normal state
11. _____osis; failure of ossification
12. Longitudinal collection of nerve fibers in the brain
13. _____uria; normal urine flow
21. Hydroxyethyl starch (abbrev.)
22. _____ation; protrusion of a structure
25. _____ceptor; pain detector
26. _____ism; coitus interruptus
27. _____algia; tooth pain
28. _____cide; an agent that destroys mosquitoes
29. Angiotensin receptor blocker (abbrev.)
31. _____algia; breast pain
32. Otoacoustic emission (abbrev.)
33. Protective plaster shell
34. A looplike structure
35. _____osis; falling out of the hair
37. Referring to a charged particle
38. Digital subtraction angiography (abbrev.)
39. Done for the sake of appearance
43. _______dynia; tongue pain
44. Main protein found in milk
45. ____ectomy; excision of a bone
46. _____oncus; tumor of the lip
47. _____gogue; producing watery discharge
48. _____iform; Y-shaped, U-shaped
49. A suspensory device
50. Prefix denoting five
52. _____phobia; fear of traveling
53. _____toe; hallux varus
54. Behavior pattern individuals present to others
55. Not obstructed
56. A complete bend in a vessel forming a circular ring

Across

1. Islet cell antibody (abbrev.)
4. Warms
9. A small bottle
13. A sound of distinct frequency
15. Beginning
16. ____genesis; origin and growth of a neoplasm
17. Continuous positive airway pressure (abbrev.)
18. Large, back chewing tooth
19. ____ually; toward the tongue
20. Excision of half of the stomach
23. Denature
24. ___sarcosis; a muscular articulation
25. ______cephaly; wedge-shaped head
28. To salute with the lips
30. An___ysm; blood vessel bulge
33. The mentum
34. Joint type at atlas and axis
35. Prefix meaning 'before'
36. A morbid concern about one's own health
40. Inosine triphosphate (abbrev.)
41. _____ alba; white line
42. ____agious; communicable
43. ___phobia; fear of animals
44. Expanded disability status scale (abbrev.)
45. Segmented median part of the cerebellum
47. Glomerular filtration rate (abbrev.)
48. Cells that produce insulin
49. A malignant tumor of the liver
57. ____lary; referring to the armpit
58. _____algia; body pain
59. Fe
60. Behavior pattern individuals present to others
61. _____malacia; softening of the iris
62. Atherosclerotic cardiovascular disease (abbrev.)
63. To breathe (suffix)
64. _____iasis; male hypersexuality
65. Referring to a female

Down

1. Scratch trigger
2. Overcome
3. ____nestic; assisting the memory
4. ______cephalus; having a flattened head
5. _____osis; bone mass within a bone
6. Antistreptolysin-O test (abbrev.)
7. Lacrimal gland secretion
8. A force that threatens homeostasis
9. Electromotive force units
10. ____pagus; twins joined at the occiput
11. American College of Nuclear Medicine (abbrev.)
12. The study or science of (suffix)
14. _______rrhagia; prolonged menstruation
21. Prefix meaning "to become or produce"
22. _____tis; inflammation of the urinary bladder
25. _____encephaly; division of the brain tissues
26. _____medicine; herbal medicine
27. _____cratic Oath; physicians oath
28. _____thesia; the sensation of muscle movements
29. Intravenous drug abuse (abbrev.)
30. Bath salt
31. _____ferous; Conveying urine
32. Relaxes
34. 'Bridge' between the medulla and the midbrain
37. Partially split or divided
38. The production and excretion of sweat
39. Congenital absence of the skull
45. A pathogen transmitting organism
46. ___ology; study of disease causes
47. A helmet-shaped structure
48. Prefix meaning 'slow'
49. ____axophobia; fear of robbers
50. Protein synthesis coding region of DNA
51. An individual hemorrhoidal tumor
52. ____coid; scapular process
53. ____osis; direct nuclear division
54. ____itis; inflammation of the testis
55. To change in position
56. ____ology; study of men's health

13

Across

1. ____algia; burning pain
5. A small outgrowth or polyp
8. Basic units of living things
13. American College of Nuclear Physicians (abbrev.)
14. ____dynia; labor pains
15. _____thymia; inability to describe one's emotions
16. Cauda
17. ____cent; moving from
18. Enzyme released by the kidney
19. Narrowing of an artery
22. Prefix meaning 'one billionth'
23. ___bus; border or margin
24. Negatively charged ions
27. Abbreviation for intrauterine device
29. ____genesis; the formation of gas
33. Not fluid
34. _____pyesis; suppuration in bone
36. Bloodshot
37. Incision of the sclera and iris
40. U.S. doctors gp.
41. Dura _____; outer brain and spinal cord membrane
42. An organic substance, insoluble in water
43. Specific sites
45. Louse egg
46. ______gastria; absence of a stomach opening
47. ___ology; study of nonliving things
49. ____nestic; assisting the memory
50. Inflammation of the stomach and intestines
58. _____phobia; fear of public places
59. Injure
60. ____ambulic; pertaining to sleepwalking
61. Referring to a charged particle
62. ____tropic; directed against the cause
63. Dull, steady pain
64. _____oid; pulley-shaped
65. Abbreviation for cathode ray oscilloscope
66. A complete bend in a vessel forming a circular ring

Down

1. ____menia; menstruation
2. ____ology; study of mites and ticks
3. One of the components of a whole
4. Resembling the spleen
5. Restricted, prohibited, or forbidden
6. Adult respiratory distress syndrome (abbrev.)
7. Condition associated with excessive uric acid
8. _____vore; meat-eater
9. Oil tumor
10. Focusing device
11. Roman sixty-two
12. Breaks religious or moral laws
14. Aches
20. Governed by chance
21. Older person
24. _____ism; absence of saliva
25. _____cyte; healthy red blood cell
26. _____ crest; pelvic ridge
27. A small cluster of cells
28. ____itis; inflammation in the womb
30. Irregularly notched, toothed, or indented
31. To become less severe for a time
32. _____meter; pain measuring instrument
34. Prefix meaning 'eight'
35. Vessel in which substances are ground with a pestle
38. _____purulent; characterized by bloody pus
39. Final
44. Pertaining to medicine
46. _____phobia; fear of the wind
48. _____ium; arm
49. _____megaly; enlargement of an atrium
50. A manner of walking
51. ____aphobia; fear of public places
52. ____motor; related to movements caused by sound
53. Abbreviation for enterohemorrhagic Escherichia coli
54. ____emia; presence of sodium in the blood
55. ____phobia; fear of childbirth
56. ____roid; denoting a thin purulent discharge
57. A walking unit

14

Across

1. ____genic; idiopathic
5. Form into clusters
10. ____zone; drinking water sterilizer
14. ____ogy; series of 3
15. Heave
16. Blood (suffix)
17. A people
18. Affecting the extremities
19. Cripple
20. Isonicotinic acid hydrazide (abbrev.)
21. Preventing muscular spasms
23. Congenital absence of skin
25. Seized with the teeth
26. ___phthalmos; recession of the eyeball
27. Condition of equal tension
32. _____form; rib-shaped
35. Roman 107
36. ___ulus; ringlike structure
37. Inflammation of bone and cartilage
41. Had food
42. Possessive pronoun version of she
43. _____gnosis; lack of sensory recognition of a limb
44. The cutting of sinew
47. Cephalopelvic disproportion (abbrev.)
48. ___phosis; loss of the eyelashes
49. Occurring in patches
53. Denoting a circular structure
58. Early receptor potential (abbrev.)
59. Short for a shoulder muscle
60. Relaxes
61. ____itis; blood vessel inflammation
62. ____roid; resembling a dream
63. Passage leading into a cavity
64. ____cephalon; thalamus and hypothalamus
65. Costae
66. _____phobia; fear of thunderstorms
67. Treat with a light beam device

Down

1. Upper heart chambers
2. _____ mal; generalized tonic-clonic seizure
3. An indentation
4. ___oma; lipogranuloma
5. _____buccal; pertaining to head and mouth
6. Ate_____sis; collapse of lung tissue
7. ____form; shaped like a leather bottle
8. Med. school applicant's test
9. Resembling a vein
10. ______colpos; retained menstruation
11. Acute motor axonal neuropathy (abbrev.)
12. Roman 53
13. Association of American Medical Colleges (abbrev.)
21. _____rrhexis; rupture of amniotic membrane
22. Breast (slang)
24. An anatomical network
27. Bonelike tusk substance
28. Breaks moral laws
29. ____emia; presence of sodium in the blood
30. ____pagus; twins joined at the occiput
31. A looplike structure
32. Outer covering of an organ
33. ____itis; inflammation of bone
34. ____osis; a bodily passage narrowing
35. ____osis; swelling of the eye lining
38. Presence of bile in blood
39. Forces sexual intercourse
40. International Classification of Diseases (abbrev.)
45. Inflammation of the shoulder
46. Habitual spasmodic muscular movement
47. A crest
49. _____itis; blood vessel wall swelling
50. Anatomic bandlike structure
51. Impulses
52. Vertebral column
53. Smell
54. ____capsule; capsule of the kidney
55. A large flaccid vesicle
56. Focusing device
57. Antistreptolysin-O test (abbrev.)
61. Normal, everyday action (abbrev.)

15

Across

1. Critical stage of a disease

5. ____agious; communicable

9. The cheeks

14. ____ulate; to clot

15. ____itis; inflammation of the female gonad

16. _____phobia; fear of public places

17. Hereditary angioneurotic edema (acronym)

18. ____tropy; myocardial relaxation

19. _____ation; irregular skin tear

20. Excessive love of knowledge

23. Condition

24. ____ment; bone-connecting tissue

25. _____gnosis; lack of sensory recognition of a limb

29. Malayan pit viper venom

33. Chronic fatigue syndrome (abbrev.)

36. Nipples

38. A hollow cylindric structure or canal

39. Morbid fear of worms

43. ____tropic; directed against the cause

44. Unit of electrical inductance

45. VD

46. Learned drive

49. To slacken

51. Reduces a fracture

53. Sarco_____; muscle cell plasma membrane

57. Within the body

62. The terminal portion of the small intestine

63. ____robic; without oxygen

64. Bones

65. _____tis; inflammation of a nerve

66. Lower limbs between the knees and the ankles

67. ____itis; inflammation of the uterus

68. Open skin lesions

69. Regular food and liquid consumption

70. ____aly; deviation from normal

Down

1. Dull pains

2. To join together

3. Madness

4. Unabsorbed food discharged from the digestive tract

5. ____otomy; cutting operation in the vagina

6. Reproductive cell of the female

7. ____pharynx; superior portion of the pharynx

8. _____opia; perception of three images of an object

9. _______ancy; deadliness

10. ________rrhea; absence of breast milk flow

11. Specific sites

12. Part of a surface

13. Auricle

21. _____form; roof-shaped

22. ___tus; an opening

26. Kidney

27. A solemn declaration

28. _____oma; artery wall mass

30. Applies friction and pressure

31. Short for 'death notice'

32. Destitute of life

33. ____osis; swelling of the eye lining

34. ____metry; size estimation of the unborn child

35. A long, narrow opening

37. A unit of perceived loudness

40. Dampness

41. Prolactin (abbrev.)

42. _____phobia; fear of glass objects

47. Segmented median part of the cerebellum

48. 7th letter of the Greek alphabet

50. Abnormal dryness of the conjunctiva

52. Burn with hot liquid

54. _____cephalon; midbrain

55. _____dynia; breast pain

56. Fear aroused by awareness of danger

57. ____pexy; surgical fixation of ileum

58. ____algia; nerve pain

59. ____roid; resembling a dream

60. Violent anger

61. A nuisance

62. ___anity; severe mental illness

16

Across

1. ____itis; inflammation of the vagina
5. Anular flare of light surrounding a luminous body
9. _____itis; inflammation of testes sac
14. Acronym for adenosine deaminase acting on RNA
15. ____eurosis; sheet-like tendon
16. A stage in the course of development
17. Behavior pattern individuals present to others
18. ____ract; to extend forward
19. Relating to the blood
20. The making of a word to express a natural sound
23. ____thesia; lack of sensation
24. ___iculation; joint
25. ______ism; severe congenital thyroid deficiency
28. Person who does not speak
30. ___anthropy; hatred of human beings
33. The side or flank
34. ____hosis; liver disorder
35. Gut-associated lymphoid tissue (abbrev.)
36. Excessive erotic interest
39. ____section; phlebotomy
40. Endoscopic retrograde cholangiopancreatography (abbrev.)
41. _____ism; absence of saliva
42. ___genous; of the same origin
43. ____rate; soften by wetting
44. Sudden episode of illness
45. Diethyltryptamine (abbrev.)
46. A tubular passage
47. Red pigmentation of the cerebrospinal fluid
54. Speak one`s mind
55. ____brachium; forearm
56. Long, slender, flexible anatomical structure
57. _____purulent; characterized by bloody pus
58. Mark left after healing
59. Monster
60. Newborn's health test score
61. ____gram; three-dimensional image
62. Spleen

Down

1. ____tid; neck artery
2. ____toid; tooth-shaped
3. _____chezia; emotional discharge gained by uttering indecent words
4. Occurring before the proper time
5. Incomplete antigen
6. _____opia; absence of the face
7. Complete bend in a vessel forming a circular ring
8. ____geny; development of an organism
9. Globular body
10. Anterior part of the thorax
11. Nerve branches
12. Obstructive sleep apnea syndrome (abbrev.)
13. ___algia; referred pain
21. _____coria; asymmetric pupils
22. _____genic; denoting response to medical treatment
25. _____cles; collarbones
26. Forces sexual intercourse
27. Prefix referring to a race or people
28. _____genation; interbreeding of different races
29. ____osia; drinking of urine
30. Madness
31. _____ crest; pelvic ridge
32. To actively pursue or threaten a person
34. ____ular; sphincteral muscle shape
35. ________itis; inflammation of stomach and colon
37. The cessation of life
38. Dura _____; outer brain and spinal cord membrane
43. ______otropic; referring to weather-affected diseases
44. ______sclerosis; arterial wall deposit accumulation
45. Suffix meaning 'pain'
46. Pertaining to a stroke or seizure
47. Expiratory positive airway pressure (abbrev.)
48. Circular band surrounding an opening
49. A skin eruption
50. ____genesis; origin and growth of a neoplasm
51. ____lalia; pathological speech problem
52. ____versible; permanent
53. ____algia; gland pain
54. Obstructive sleep apnea (abbrev.)

17

Across

1. Big, clumsy people
5. Restores to health
10. ____naceous; soapy
14. A dose of medicine
15. Prefix meaning 'head'
16. ____otomy; incision into an apical structure
17. Relating to occipital bone and mastoid process
20. _____dynia; nose pain
21. To strike or tap firmly
22. White
25. ____sightedness; myopia
26. Abbreviation for dyspnea on exertion
29. Treat an anatomic structure with a light beam device
31. Stable with opposing forces in balance
35. Estrogen replacement therapy (abbrev.)
36. Prefix meaning 'within'
38. ____dynia; sinew pain
39. Dwarfism characterized by gross limb shortening and hydropic head and trunk
43. ____itis; tenosynovitis
44. _____gnosia; sensory inattention
45. Short for arm adductor
46. the odor of the axillae
49. Toward the mouth
50. ___pose; fatty
51. ____insic; of internal origin
53. ____eurosis; sheet-like tendon
55. Dies
58. Pertaining to sound
62. Stimulating to secretion
65. A manner of walking
66. Whiteheads
67. ____osis; direct nuclear division
68. ____mania; compulsive shopping
69. _____omosis; blood vessel coalescence
70. A small round structure

Down

1. Smell
2. Superior aortic curve
3. Central points
4. _____ bifida; vertebral arch fusion failure
5. Hydrochloric acid (abbrev.)
6. Consume
7. ____tosis; cell suicide
8. The external opening of a space
9. Looks intently
10. Soak
11. ____taxis; slight hemorrhage
12. Bony landmark located below PSIS
13. Obsessive-compulsive disorder (abbrev.)
18. ______osis; hay fever
19. ____emia; intestinal autointoxication
23. ____age; dressing holder
24. _____phobia; fear of thunderstorms
26. The cessation of life
27. _____algia; pain in the testes
28. Used as an early anaesthetic
30. _____genic; causing sexual arousal
32. SI unit of magnetic flux density
33. In a direction toward the inion
34. _____form; rib-shaped
37. _____phobia; fear of public places
40. Prefix referring to the back of the head
41. Expiratory positive airway pressure (abbrev.)
42. Having many projections or protuberances
47. A component of a whole
48. Supporting framework of an organ
52. An organic substance, insoluble in water
54. _____encephalia; absence of the cerebellum
55. ____thropic; originating outside the human body
56. Roman 92
57. ____phobia; fear of light flashes
59. ____topic; occurring at the usual place
60. ____ectomy; surgical removal of part of the iris
61. Suffix meaning 'cell'
62. The self
63. Abbreviation for carcinoma in situ
64. Disease-spreading rodent

1	2	3	4	■	5	6	7	8	■	9	10	11	12	13
14				■	15				■	16				
17				18					19					
20					■	■	21							
22					23	24	■	25			■	■	■	■
■	■	■	■	■	26		27			■	28	29	30	31
32	33	34	35	36				■	■	37				
38								39	40					
41					■	■	42							
43				■	44	45				■	■	■	■	■
■	■	■	■	46			■	47		48	49	50	51	52
53	54	55	56				57	■	■	58				
59								60	61					
62					■	63				■	64			
65					■	66				■	67			

Across

1. ____form; xiphoid
5. ____ology; study of mites and ticks
9. Marks left after healing
14. Decays
15. Biological unit of heredity
16. Head
17. Study of diseases of the nails
20. _____phobia; fear of being buried alive
21. Anterior to a kidney
22. Pertaining to dreaming
25. Suffix meaning 'enzyme'
26. Prefix meaning 'heart'
28. ____coid; scapular process
32. A lymph reservoir
37. Instrument used to lift or pry
38. Between vertebral pedicles
41. Odor
42. Equality in the size of the two pupils
43. ____phobia; fear of certain places
44. A sonorous and convulsive inspiration
46. Prefix meaning 'less'
47. Recurring every third day
53. Toward the head
58. _____schisis; cleft palate
59. Dwarfism characterized by gross limb shortening and hydropic head and trunk
62. _____form; cartwheel-patterned
63. ____osis; a bodily passage narrowing
64. Act out with gestures and body movement
65. Amyo_____; muscle tone defect
66. Eye, ear, nose, and throat (abbrev.)
67. Obstructive sleep apnea syndrome (abbrev.)

Down

1. _____genic; causing sexual arousal
2. Occurring on the ninth day
3. A tampon
4. _____algia; sciatica
5. Gone by
6. Congenital erythropoietic porphyria (abbrev.)
7. Anionic neutrophil-activating peptide (abbrev.)
8. Toward the back part
9. Numerical evaluation of achievement
10. ____facient; substance that warms
11. ____eurosis; sheet-like tendon
12. A mucous membrane fold
13. ____oid; pencil-like
18. ___mone; bodily secretion
19. ____tancy; an involuntary delay
23. International Commission on Radiological Protection (abbrev.)
24. Walking stick
27. Transmitter or receiver
28. Abbreviation for chicken embryo lethal orphan (virus)
29. ____itis; inflammation of the female gonad
30. ____form; resembling a network
31. Part of a surface
32. ____tern; reservoir
33. ____ordination; ataxia
34. Walking unit
35. ____dynia; sinew pain
36. Estrogen replacement therapy (abbrev.)
37. ___idity; clearness of thought
39. ____onic; having equal tension
40. Overcome
44. Living in a natural state
45. Having a noisy voice
46. Madness
48. Move swiftly on foot
49. _____phobia; fear of involuntarily shaking
50. Suffix meaning 'a disease process resulting therefrom'
51. The soul or life
52. Olfactory organs
53. Protective plaster shell
54. ____genous; originating outside the organism
55. Unit of apparent loudness
56. ____zontal; perpendicular to the vertical
57. Anti____; poison-stopping substance
60. ___eric; nonproprietary
61. Abbreviation for ears, nose, and throat

19

Across

1. ____itis; inflammation of a bone
5. Grows older
9. Pertaining to birds
14. ____osis; swelling of the eye lining
15. ____osis; state of stupor
16. Auricle
17. A shade of a color
18. Muscular action induced by a dominant idea
20. In a direction toward the inion
22. _____ectomy; excision of the skull
23. Drools
26. Treat an anatomic structure with a light beam device
30. Like a wing
31. Pertaining to the backbone
33. Clinical Laboratory Assistant (abbrev.)
36. A fetus with only a rudimentary body
39. _____phobia; fear of public places
40. Heavy pigmentation of the liver
43. Speak one`s opinion without fear or hesitation
44. The soul or life
45. ___ology; metaphysical study of the nature of being and existence
46. A small hollow
48. A sudden, sharp spasm of pain
50. A dose of medicine
51. Medulla _________
56. Spiral in form
58. The terminal portion of the small intestine
60. Superior to an artery
65. ____tive; purgative
66. Prefix meaning 'head'
67. A measure of duration
68. Obstructive sleep apnea syndrome (abbrev.)
69. A just detectable amount
70. ____ocratic Oath; physicians oath
71. ____atomic; denoting five atoms per molecule

Down

1. Prefix meaning 'eight'
2. Anterior legs
3. Any anatomic bandlike structure
4. Emergency Medical Treatment and Labor Act (abbrev.)
5. ___lingus; sexual stimulation of the anus
6. Abbreviation for glutamate decarboxylase
7. Vertical in position
8. Numerical evaluation of achievement
9. ____eurosis; sheet-like tendon
10. Acquired leukoderma
11. ___encephaly; occipital cranial defect, with brain exposed
12. ___dontia; absence of teeth
13. ___ism; dwarfishness
19. A quantity of matter
21. Expands or swells
24. ____constriction; narrowing of blood vessels
25. An agreeable odor
27. _____gnosia; denial of a neurological deficit
28. Used as a nerve gas in chemical warfare
29. _____osis; degeneration of collagen fibers
32. _______itis; inflammation of all blood vessel coats
33. Ligament, tendon or band of fibrous tissue
34. A person with Hansen disease
35. _____lysis; surgical collapse of the apex of the lung
37. Adult males
38. _____tropic; not effecting fat metabolism
41. Without kidneys
42. Acute motor axonal neuropathy (abbrev.)
47. Plantar surface of the foot
49. A triple cadence to the heart sounds
52. Process of being born
53. Roman sixty-three
54. To tantalize
55. _____ology; study of growth
57. Feminine suffix
59. ____algia; breast pain
60. Abbreviation for electroconvulsive therapy
61. ___amnesia; false recollection
62. U.S. psychiatrists' gp.
63. Adenosine monophosphate (abbrev.)
64. ___idic; pertaining to scales

Across

1. Clinical Laboratory Improvement Amendments (abbrev.)
5. _____ferous; yielding milk
10. Abbreviation for inosine triphosphate
13. ____brain; rhombencephalon
14. _____phobia; fear of public places
15. ____phobia; fear of different mental conceptions
16. Within the peritoneal cavity
19. Prefix meaning 'smooth'
20. A narrow passage
21. A flat structure or layer
22. A unit of brightness
24. The back of the feet
25. ____psoas; hip flexor
26. Having little height
28. To close an ion channel
30. _____phobia; fear of small skin parasites
31. 21st letter of the Greek alphabet
34. Vitamin B2 deficiency
38. Foot
39. Abnormalities indicative of disease
40. Openings or foramina
41. 1st cervical vertebra
42. ____ture; an opening
44. Uterus
46. Pertaining to the skull
49. An indentation
50. _____form; cartwheel-patterned
52. U.S. doctors gp.
53. Regeneration of bone
56. Mark left after healing
57. Aches
58. Nore____phrine; a neurotransmitter
59. ___algia; referred pain
60. Bifurcated
61. ____rhea; maintenance of water equilibrium

Down

1. A cold, shivering sensation
2. Line
3. Inflammation of the innermost layer
4. Adverse drug reaction (abbrev.)
5. ______myitis; inflammation of the abdominal muscles
6. Active substance capable of producing an effect
7. ____coid; scapular process
8. ____ogy; series of three
9. ___rology; the science of medicine
10. A standard of perfection
11. Nipples
12. Either extremity of any axis
15. A passage leading into a cavity
17. Angiotensin-converting enzyme inhibitors (abbrev.)
18. Genetic functional unit controlling production of a messenger RNA
23. A large flaccid vesicle
24. ____zontal; perpendicular to the vertical
26. Examines with a sensing device
27. Hand arm vibration syndrome (abbrev.)
28. A communicating junction
29. ___flexia; lack of reflexes
30. Seaweed
31. Chronic, non-contagious skin disease
32. ___cus; axillae odor
33. International sensitivity index (abbrev.)
35. ______toxism; poisoning from eating contaminated oysters
36. Structures of threadlike appearance
37. Not obstructed
41. _____oma; artery wall mass
42. To stop
43. Ache
44. _____genation; interbreeding of different races
45. Situated on the outside
46. _____tion; the process of knowing
47. _____ acid; protein part
48. Light beam device
49. ____algia; homesickness
50. A short sharp sound
51. Cauda
54. Adenosine 5-phosphosulfate (abbrev.)
55. Prefix meaning 'upon' or 'above'

21

Across

1. ____emia; blood volume deficiency
5. Affected with madness
10. Control of Communicable Diseases Manual (abbrev.)
14. ____genesis; reproduction by segmentation
15. _____dynia; pain in a gland
16. Prefix meaning 'oil'
17. ____aly; deviation from normal
18. Graft
20. Left
22. _____kinesis; movement in the body tissues
23. Puberty person
24. _______rhea; mucous discharge from the anus
26. Protein-covered globules of cholesterol
30. Mature person
31. Extracorporeal membrane oxygenation (abbrev.)
32. Human leukocyte antigens (abbrev.)
35. Prefix referring to 'eyelash'
36. Enzyme-linked immunosorbent assay (abbrev.)
38. Ache
39. ___ology; regional anatomy
40. ____otomy; incision into an apical structure
41. Carcino_____; cancer-producing
42. Headache
45. _______dynia; chest pain
49. Protective cover on the dorsal distal phalanx
50. _____acusis; excessive sensitivity to sound
51. Relating to the an organ's outer layer
55. Surgical cut made during childbirth
58. ____otomy; cutting operation in the vagina
59. ____agious; communicable
60. _____opsia; visual perseveration
61. Prefix meaning 'lip'
62. ____thesia; lack of sensation
63. Forefinger
64. ____tropic; directed against the cause

Down

1. Tumors (suffix)
2. ____tive; a demulcent remedy
3. Fe
4. Intricately coiled and looped capillary vessels
5. Anything that occupies space and has mass
6. ______genic; of suprarenal origin
7. ____sightedness; myopia
8. ___ocuous; harmless
9. Chief of Staff (abbrev.)
10. Severe abdominal pain causing crying
11. Osteo_____; bone tissue resorbing cell
12. _____alveolitis; periodontal disease
13. Muscle contraction neuron
19. _____phobia; fear of one's own voice
21. ____icemia; blood poisoning
24. Short for chest muscles
25. A cleft or crack
26. ____ose; milk sugar
27. ____pathic; of unknown origin
28. Soft innermost layer of a tooth
29. _____opsia; migraine aura
32. ____nail; fingernail root skin
33. Roman 53
34. Antineutrophil cytoplasmic antibodies (abbrev.)
36. Enteropathogenic Escherichia coli (abbrev.)
37. ____philia; a liking for fats
38. A thin skin or film
40. _____cide; mite-destroying agent
41. A manner of walking
43. Absence or weakening of social norms or values
44. Voice-box
45. A capsule or sheath
46. _____oia; sluggish mental activity
47. Speak one`s opinion without fear or hesitation
48. Relaxes
51. Having a uncomfortably lower than normal temperature
52. The outer covering of an organ
53. ____cans; becoming white
54. ____myosarcoma; malignant tumor of the uterus muscle
56. ___oid; morphine-like
57. Brownish skin colour

22

Across

1. _____cyte; fat cell
6. Part of a surface
10. Of sound mind
14. _____rrhea; drooling
15. To breathe rapidly and shallowly
16. ____oid; lens-shaped
17. A sudden attack
18. Conjoined twins in which the bodies are joined laterally
20. Suture of the aorta
22. A benign neoplasm of muscular tissue
23. Fetal attitude
24. ___era; rough
27. Tunica _____; middle artery wall layer
30. The shin
32. The cheek
35. ____ology; the science of medicine
37. A compound of oxygen with another element or a radical
38. Not obstructed
39. Between (prefix)
41. ____rysm; blood vessel dilation
42. An ounce
44. Motion picture
45. ____osis; exaggerated lumbar curve
46. _______genous; causing lockjaw
48. To join together
50. Hepatitis-associated antigen (abbrev.)
51. Inosine 5-monophosphate (abbrev.)
53. A holding device
56. Tissue grafting
60. Spur-shaped
63. _____mesis; vomiting of saliva
64. C2
65. Enteric cytopathogenic swine orphan (abbrev.)
66. Small, congenital, pigmented, skin spots
67. The soft inner substance of a hair
68. The ratio of output to input of an amplifying system
69. _____omosis; blood vessel coalescence

Down

1. Ab____; inability to walk
2. Digital Imaging and Communications in Medicine (abbrev.)
3. Medical practice specialty (suffix)
4. An abnormal craving for wealth
5. A cytoplasmic body in the ovum that passes into the germ cell
6. ____ture; an opening
7. ____itis; inflammation of the vertebral column
8. Inner
9. Referring to an allergic reaction in the skin
10. To remove the ovaries of an animal
11. Antihemophilic globulin (abbrev.)
12. ___pathia; seasickness
13. Electrocerebral silence (abbrev.)
19. _____type ; the observed properties of a trait
21. Lateral forearm bones
24. _____ acid; protein part
25. _____osis, hyperferremia
26. _____esthesia; phantom limb pain
28. International Anatomical Nomenclature Committee (abbrev.)
29. Epitympanic recess
31. An utterance of joy
32. The oral cavity
33. Absence of autonomic breathing
34. Ate_____sis; collapse of lung tissue
36. ____genic; originating in the kidney
40. Respond to a stimulus
43. The soul or life
47. ______nate; to fertilize
49. Clear, yellowish fluid portion of blood
52. A fold
54. _____denitis; salivary gland inflammation
55. The extremities of any axis
56. Interstitial cell-stimulating hormone (abbrev.)
57. ____form; loop-shaped
58. An inert gaseous element in the atmosphere
59. A small mass of foreign cells
60. Cradle ___; infant scalp disease
61. ___fugal; extending away from a center line
62. ___mus; acidity or alkalinity indicator

23

Across

1. HIV/AIDS reporting system (acronym)
5. Numerical evaluation of achievement
10. Excitatory postsynaptic potential (abbrev.)
14. Enteropathogenic Escherichia coli (abbrev.)
15. Any wasting of the body
16. Cns 'matter' consisting of nonmyelinated nerve tissue
17. ____itis; inflammation of the uterus
18. To discharge waste
19. ____blast; nucleus of the fertilized oocyte
20. Loss of sensation of the extremities
23. Nipples
24. Enteroinvasive Escherichia coli (abbrev.)
25. Computed tomography angiography (abbrev.)
27. Deviating from what is ordinary
28. Female breast (slang)
31. Muscle contraction neuron
33. ________pathy; ill health due to climate
37. Residue remaining after percolation of a drug
38. Abnormally large brain
41. Antineutrophil cytoplasmic antibodies (abbrev.)
42. Turns around an axis
43. ______brae; spinal segments
45. Abbreviation for dead on arrival
46. Prefix meaning 'below'
49. Certified Medical Assistant (abbrev.)
50. Oscitate
54. ______cephalus; small-headed person
56. ______________osis; hardening of the brain
60. _____pagus; twins joined at the occiput
61. A ripe ovum
62. Prefix signifying one trillion
63. _____esis; urine increase
64. ______valgus; flattened and outward turned longitudinal foot arch
65. Acute necrotizing ulcerative gingivitis (abbrev.)
66. Enteric cytopathogenic swine orphan (abbrev.)
67. ______cephalon; endbrain
68. The measured quantity of a drug

Down

1. _______colpos; retained menstruation
2. Autoimmune polyendocrinopathy-candidiasis-ectodermal dystrophy (abbrev.)
3. Toward the back part
4. ______itis; inflammation of the testes sac
5. _____osis; a bodily passage narrowing
6. Rib ____; skeletal thorax
7. Excessively overweight
8. ______form; ropelike
9. An_______sia; lack of normal sensation
10. Ova
11. Occurring before a stroke, seizure or attack
12. Conducive to health
13. ___genic; producing pus
21. ______oid; resembling a star
22. Erythema chronicum migrans (abbrev.)
26. AIDS-related complex (abbrev.)
29. A tubular passage
30. ____dynia; sinew pain
32. Tumors (suffix)
33. Med. school applicant's test
34. Optic coherence tomography (abbrev.)
35. To see and understand words
36. ___kinetic; pertaining to eye movement
38. Relating to memory
39. A malformed fetus having no skull
40. Restores to health
41. Atrioventricular conduction (abbrev.)
44. Oculus
46. ______dynia; pain in the spleen
47. Womb
48. GLA-rich medicinal herb
51. ______osis; cell suicide
52. Complete
53. Pertaining to birth
55. Outward
57. ____meter; pupillometer
58. Narrow elevation of a bone
59. ____toid; tooth-shaped
60. ___ology; science of the development mental conceptions

1	2	3	4	■	5	6	7	8	■	9	10	11	12	13
14				■	15				■	16				
17				■	18				■	19				
20				21					22					■
■	■	■	■	23			■	24				■	■	■
25	26	27	28			■	29				■	30	31	32
33					■	34				■	35			
36					37					38				
39				■	40				■	41				
42			■	43				■	44					
■	■	■	45				■	46			■	■	■	■
■	47	48					49				50	51	52	53
54					■	55				■	56			
57					■	58				■	59			
60					■	61				■	62			

Across

1. Hollow spaces
5. Uniformly advancing disturbance in which the parts undergo a double oscillation
9. _____phobia; fear of thunderstorms
14. Acute motor axonal neuropathy (abbrev.)
15. Grows older
16. To dye
17. Treat an anatomic structure with a light beam device
18. ____motor; related to movements caused by sound
19. Concave parts of the hands
20. Fear of closed spaces
23. Carcinoembryonic antigen (abbrev.)
24. Not his
25. Anal injections of fluid
29. _____phobia; fear of certain places
30. Adeno-associated virus (abbrev.)
33. Not general or systemic
34. ____coid; scapular 'process'
35. Antineutrophil cytoplasmic antibodies (abbrev.)
36. Within the peritoneal cavity
39. ____ology; anatomy of the soft parts of the body
40. ____gonist; agonist's opposer
41. _____feric; increasing sodium transport
42. ___dontia; absence of teeth
43. ____culus; joint
44. Resembling a cell
45. Spiked projection from a bone
46. ___cyx; tailbone
47. Suture of an artery
54. The lower inner surface of a hollow organ
55. Toward the mouth
56. ____robic; without oxygen
57. To end a pregnancy
58. ____ment; liquid preparation rubbed into the skin
59. ____phobia; fear of light flashes
60. Expression of the quantity of a substance in relation to another
61. suffix meaning 'condition'
62. Pilus

Down

1. ____aneus; heel bone
2. ____gam; cavity filler
3. Vessels
4. ____rysm; blood vessel dilation
5. Decays
6. _____phobia; fear of public places
7. ____fibrosis; phlebosclerosis
8. Tendency for the eyes to turn inward
9. ______genous; not producing spores
10. Pierces with a pointed instrument
11. ____pedic; clubfooted
12. A cleft or crack
13. Autonomic nervous system (abbrev.)
21. A stairlike structure
22. _____itis; inflammation of the liver
25. Enzyme-linked immunosorbent assay (abbrev.)
26. Occurring on the ninth day
27. _____geny; absence or defect of any bodily part
28. Residue remaining after percolation of a drug
29. _____pelvis; twisted pelvis
30. _____derma; looseness and atrophy of the skin
31. _____cide; mite-destroying agent
32. Verifiably correct
34. Cylindrical structure within a centrosome
35. ____omy; body structure study
37. _____esis; inhibited urination
38. _____itis; inflammation of the nails
43. ______gnathia; open bite
44. Of the heart
45. ____ form; cartwheel-patterned
46. _____ectomy; excision of the skull
47. White
48. Lowermost attaching structure
49. Fetor ____; halitosis
50. Adrenal androgen-stimulating hormone (abbrev.)
51. To breathe (suffix)
52. ____phagia; ingestion of an excessive quantity of salts
53. The time the earth takes to revolve around the sun
54. ___ sight; hyperopia

25

Across

1. Pertaining to birds
6. A chill or fit of shivering
10. Round, flat anatomical structure
14. Decompression sickness
15. ____ular; sphincteral muscle shape
16. Ethylenediaminetetraacetic acid (acronym)
17. Within the peritoneal cavity
20. Otoacoustic emission (acronym)
21. Instrumental activities of daily living (acronym)
22. Any medication containing opium
23. Lateral forearm bones
25. Prefix meaning 'over a distance'
26. Other licensed antifungal therapies (acronym)
28. Inflammation of a nerve branch
32. A spot or blemish
34. ____itis; inflammation of an apex
35. Anodal closure contraction (acronym)
38. Between the metatarsal bones
42. Carcinoma in situ (acronym)
43. A people
44. _____cephalus; small-headed person
45. Relating to heat
48. Nipple
49. Warmth
51. Prefix meaning 'above' or 'beyond'
53. Pertaining to the urinary bladder
55. ____otomy; cutting operation in the vagina
56. ___phosis; loss of the eyelashes
59. Pertaining to the optic nerve and pupil
62. ____meter; pupillometer
63. ____aria; heat rash
64. Medical Latin term for mild
65. ____eurosis; sheet-like tendon
66. ____gonist; agonist's opposer
67. _____gnosia; denial of a neurological deficit

Down

1. ____genesis; development of life from nonlife
2. ____ cava; main vein
3. Influences each other
4. Adverse drug reaction (acronym)
5. Non-steroidal anti-inflammatory drug (acronym)
6. Condition of listlessness and a form of melancholia
7. Female youth
8. ___nation; micturation
9. ____genous; originating outside the organism
10. Refuses to admit
11. A standard of perfection
12. A condition
13. ____facient; substance that warms
18. Two objects considered together because of similarity
19. Pertaining to vision
24. ____roma; artery wall mass
26. Aural
27. ____ary; adapted for tearing
29. Dura _____; outer brain and spinal cord membrane
30. Isopropyl alcohol (acronym)
31. Breast (slang)
33. Having no fixed or regular course
35. _________genic; failing in sperm production
36. ____menia; menstruation
37. End result of coagulation
39. Grand ___; generalized tonic-clonic seizure
40. Prefix meaning 'habitat'
41. An anatomical network
45. A positively charged ion
46. Equality of vision in both eyes
47. ____cide; an agent that destroys mosquitoes
49. _____epsia; impaired digestion
50. Prefix referring a female hormone
52. The under surface of the foot
53. The source of cocaine
54. Brain state of total unresponsiveness to all external stimuli
55. A system of extreme religious beliefs and rituals
57. Rainbow-like eye part
58. Dissolution (prefix)
60. A metallic bone implant
61. ___itis; inflammation of gastric cellular tissue

26

Across

1. Inhibitory postsynaptic potential (acronym)
5. A delimited area
10. Prefix meaning 'eight'
14. ____opia; double vision
15. Assigns a category
16. ____coid; scapular process
17. Winglike structures
18. Active substance capable of producing an effect
19. ____oris; erectile female organ
20. Between two joints
23. The back of the foot
24. A disease or illness
25. Stupid people
28. Highly active antiretroviral therapy (abbrev.)
30. To turn outward
31. _____alveolitis; periodontal disease
32. ___iotic; fluid surrounding the fetus
35. ____tic; mentally ill person
36. A salt of uric acid
37. Prefix meaning 'oil'
38. ___dynia; shoulder pain
39. _____form; cartwheel-patterned
40. Ilio_____; thigh flexor
41. Walking units
42. Open or exposed
43. A basic garment for infants
46. Either extremity of any axis
47. Relating to the occipital bone and C1
52. ____algia; nose pain
53. SI unit of magnetic flux density
54. ____dotal; based on case histories
56. A unit of perceived loudness
57. _____itis; inflammation of the innermost layer
58. ____ceptor; free nerve ending that detects pain
59. Fetor ____; halitosis
60. _____cephaly; narrowness of the head
61. Lateral attachment of inguinal ligament (abbrev.)

Down

1. Iminodiacetate (acronym)
2. Hairs
3. The full extent of anything
4. An excess of any of the body fluids
5. Looks intently
6. Relating to the buttocks
7. ____ture; an opening
8. ____rum; middle of body
9. A rough calculation
10. Obscured or concealed
11. _____genosis; connectve tissue disease
12. A group of three associated entities
13. Medical practice specialty (suffix)
21. Eye, ear, nose, and throat (acronym)
22. ____tid; neck artery
25. ____mania; abnormal liking for music
26. Female reproductive
27. ____genic; originating in the kidney
28. Perceives by the ears
29. Prefix meaning 'against'
31. A dose of medicine
32. Plant derived juice used on skin
33. Average
34. ____algia; homesickness
36. Inflammation in the womb
37. _______genesis; bone regeneration
39. Walking unit
40. ____esthesia; perception of vibration
41. Vertebral columns
42. ______phobia; fear of rivers
43. _____dynia; back pain
44. A thin serous discharge from a wound
45. Alveoli
46. _____opsia; visual perseveration
48. A bed covering for administering oxygen
49. ____itis; inflammation of a bone
50. ____emia; excess fibrin in the blood
51. ____bel; loudness measurement unit
55. Carcinoma in situ (acronym)

27

Across

1. Away from the surface
5. To draw or force liquids or gases
9. _____gnosia; sensory inattention
14. Insect parasite that causes scabies
15. The sum of all instincts for self-preservation
16. _____rhea; excessive menstruation
17. Sperm
18. Prefix meaning 'one billionth'
19. _____phobia; fear of thunderstorms
20. Relating to occipital bone and mastoid process
23. ____facient; substance that warms
24. Prefix meaning 'eight'
25. Fully developed
28. ______blast; a tissue-forming cell
32. Deficient in active properties
33. _____ aponeurotica; epicranial aponeurosis
36. ___nism; coitus interruptus
37. Masculine
38. Decompression sickness
39. Material from which the glaze for artificial teeth is made
40. Internal Mammary Artery (acronym)
41. A narrow passage
42. A pathologic startle syndrome
43. The shin
45. Imitates
46. Ab____; inability to walk
48. _____lalia; pathological speech problem
49. Facial neuralgia caused by a decayed tooth
56. ______icular; relating to a heart chamber
57. Sodium chloride
58. Infraorbitomeatal line (acronym)
59. ______genic; starch-forming
60. _____culus; joint
61. Acute necrotizing ulcerative gingivitis (acronym)
62. The external opening of a space
63. Enur____; urinary incontinence
64. Treat an anatomic structure with a light beam device

Down

1. Dimethyl sulfoxide (acronym)
2. Enteroinvasive Escherichia coli (acronym)
3. Enterotoxigenic Escherichia coli (acronym)
4. Care and treatment of the feet
5. Relating to the male copulatory organ
6. A salt of uric acid
7. ____plegia; paralysis of one limb
8. _____phagia; swallowing food without thorough mastication
9. Absence of one or more mammary glands
10. The male gonad
11. ____geny; development of an organism
12. Openings or foramina
13. Toward the mouth
21. A portion
22. Dull pains
25. To imitate or simulate
26. ______esis; recollection
27. Weblike tissues
29. ______pelvis; twisted pelvis
30. Relating to the inion
31. Solemn declarations
33. ___eric; nonproprietary
34. ___biosis; resuscitation
35. The bad cholesterol (acronym)
38. Prefix referring to a foundation
39. Tending to occur in a household
41. A segment of DNA equivalent to a gene
42. ____ment; bone-connecting tissue
44. A covering layer
45. Rigor ______; muscular stiffening following death
47. Looplike structures
48. Prefix meaning 'many'
49. Egg shaped
50. Prefix meaning 'half'
51. Prefix meaning 'name'
52. Hearing organs
53. ____duct; seminal duct or uterine tube
54. Most inferior of several similar structures
55. ____sthesia; pain sense

Across

1. ____tectomy; removal of the liver

5. ____atomic; denoting five atoms per molecule

9. Acute motor axonal neuropathy (acronym)

13. Smallest unit of an element

14. _____phobia; fear of small skin parasites

16. _____plegia; paralysis of one limb

17. Turned toward the median plane

19. ____encephalon; forebrain

20. ______ectasis; vasodilation of the arteries

21. Consume

22. Organism in or on which a parasite lives

23. Brainstem auditory evoked potential (acronym)

25. _______phobia; fear of old people

27. A device for estimating the sensitivity to odorants

31. ___cardia; systole

32. ____dynia; sinew pain

33. To imitate or simulate

37. Anionic neutrophil-activating peptide (acronym)

39. Pertaining to sound

42. Chicken embryo lethal orphan (acronym)

43. Male ejaculatory fluid

45. Active range of motion (acronym)

47. ___ital; of a finger

48. Harmonization

52. Milk sugar

55. Of sound mind

56. ____phia; a wasting away

57. To elicit a tendon reflex

59. To touch so as to cause laughter

63. Lacrimal gland secretion

64. The process of wasting away of the body

66. Medial forearm bone

67. _____dynia; pain in the uterus

68. One of the components of a whole

69. Dirt

70. ____algia; nose pain

71. ____rrhagia; excessive uterine bleeding

Down

1. Human antimouse antibody (abbrev.)

2. ____nal; everlasting

3. Prefix meaning 'after'

4. Single-celled organism (variable)

5. Body part walls

6. Prefix meaning 'habitat'

7. The back of the neck

8. Process of sorting patients according to their need for care

9. Resembling the sound made by blowing across the neck of a bottle

10. A stupid person

11. _____osis; failure of ossification

12. _____phobia; fear of returning home

15. Group of eight

18. A passage or pathway

24. _____phobia; fear of fatigue or overworking

26. Dream state (acronym)

27. Tumors (suffix)

28. Narrow elevation of a bone

29. Small bubbles on the surface of a liquid

30. A unicellular organism

34. ____cine; science of healing

35. ____psoas; hip flexor

36. ____ition; the process of knowing

38. Pertaining to the chest

40. Rainbow-like eye part

41. An inclination

44. ___tropics; brain enhancers

46. Violent abnormal behavior

49. _____pyesis; suppuration in bone

50. A rotating tool used to enlarge holes

51. A rooflike structure

52. The side or flank

53. Prefix meaning 'incomplete'

54. _____ectomy; excision of the skull

58. ____ology; study of disease

60. ____tics; the science of motion

61. Lumbus

62. ____blast; a cell nucleolus

65. ___coid; ring-shaped

1	2	3	4	■	5	6	7	8	9	■	10	11	12	13
14				■	15					■	16			
17				18						■	19			
■	■	20			■	■	21			■	22			
■	23				24	25				26				
27							■	■	28			■	■	■
29			■	30			31	32	■	33		34	35	36
37			38	■	39				40	■	41			
42				43	■	44				45	■	46		
■	■	■	47		48	■	■	49			50			
51	52	53				54	55							■
56				■	57			■	■	58			■	■
59				■	60			61	62				63	64
65				■	66					■	67			
68				■	69					■	70			

Across

1. Incapable of normal locomotion
5. A two-footed conjoined twin
10. International Classification of Diseases (acronym)
14. ____tia; denoting lack of force
15. Deficient in active properties
16. A spiral
17. Innermost heart wall layers
19. ____ital; health care institution
20. Iminodiacetate (acronym)
21. American College of Radiology (acronym)
22. ____itis; inflammation of the testis
23. Congenital absence of the head and heart
27. The act of avoiding
28. Hypothetical mean organism (acronym)
29. Costa
30. _____rhea; excessive talking
33. A flat, fluid-filled sac
37. ____facient; substance that warms
39. _____ography; muscle and organ movement recording
41. Reduces a fracture
42. _____atic; relating to gas or air
44. Group of eight
46. Roman 102
47. Short for a chest muscle
49. Inspires
51. Surgical puncture and aspiration of a joint
56. ____tid; neck artery
57. Dopamine transporter (acronym)
58. Cervical intraepithelial neoplasia (acronym)
59. Like a wing
60. Inspiration
65. ____capsule; capsule of the kidney
66. Live-in child-care worker
67. ____cent; free from wrong
68. Bones
69. _____itis; inflammation of the tongue
70. Grows older

Down

1. Fetal attitude
2. ___ulus; ringlike structure
3. Treatable
4. Wears away
5. ___phragm; breathing muscle
6. International normalized ratio (acronym)
7. Relating to the feet
8. _____lysis; decomposition of uric acid
9. Amylum
10. Resembling a thin, serous wound discharge
11. _____inate; harmonize
12. Rounded, flat plates
13. 1st letter of the Greek alphabet
18. _____lary; microscopic blood vessel
23. Pertaining to birds
24. Hamulus
25. _____poiesis; blood or lymphatic vessel formation
26. ___ageusia; loss of taste on both sides of tongue
27. Endoscopic retrograde cholangiopancreatography (acronym)
31. ___ology; study of tumors
32. _____itis; inflammation of the optomeninx
34. Lying back
35. Inflammation of the sebaceous glands of the eyelids
36. Lateral attachment of inguinal ligament (abbrev.)
38. A pleasant feeling of wellbeing
40. A bed covering for administering oxygen
43. ___algia; pain in the thigh
45. A capsule or sheath
48. Translation of information into numbered categories
50. Disgust at the sight or thought of food
51. _____phobia; fear of small skin parasites
52. Bubbling sounds in the lungs
53. Prefix denoting across or through
54. a narrow passage
55. Prefix referring to a race or people
61. Autonomic nervous system (abbrev.)
62. ___emia; dissolution of red blood cells
63. A single
64. ___ophobia; fear of disease

Across

1. ____dotal; based on case histories
5. Fe
9. _____genesis; milk production
14. French for AIDS
15. _____naceous; soapy
16. _____itis; inflammation of the innermost layer
17. A tubular passage
18. Small triangular membrane formed at the caudal angle of the rhomboid fossa
19. Periodically sheds an outer covering
20. Most superficial three layers of transversospinal muscles
23. Having the disagreeable odor or taste of decomposing fats
24. Lacking normal muscle tone
28. Wing-like process
29. Prefix meaning 'with'
31. Any objective an organism seeks to attain
32. Perceive flavour in the mouth
35. Spheroid bacteria
37. Intrinsic sympathomimetic activity (acronym)
38. Narrowing of an artery
41. Computed tomography angiography (acronym)
42. _____derma; looseness and atrophy of the skin
43. Bone ridge
44. ____ditary; transmissible from parent to offspring
46. Insulin-like activity (acronym)
47. ___neous; having a woody feeling
48. Appetite
50. Inlaid
53. Producing indole
57. Anterior part of the thorax
60. ____form; resembling pus
61. ____grity; soundness of structure
62. _____phasia; abnormally rapid speech
63. Inflammation of (suffix)
64. "With no delay"
65. To tantalize
66. A sitting surface
67. ____ pubis; soft tissue bulge over the female pubes

Down

1. Lateral attachment of inguinal ligament (abbrev.)
2. Saltpeter
3. Abnormal accumulation of interstitial fluid
4. Keel-shaped
5. Equality of vision in both eyes
6. Infected with the disease of rage
7. Not obstructed
8. Anything that exerts a harmful influence
9. A boundary or end
10. ______nosia; denial of a neurological deficit
11. Cytotoxic T lymphocytes (acronym)
12. Female breast (slang)
13. Organic mood syndrome (acronym)
21. Outer layer of the eyeball
22. To incise with a sharp object
25. Unwanted sound
26. Suffix meaning 'presence of an abnormal condition or disease'
27. Osteo_____; bone tissue resorbing cell
29. A rib
30. Prefix meaning 'eight'
32. _____meter; speed measuring device
33. _____itis; blood vessel wall swelling
34. To look fixedly
35. Prefix meaning 'cavity' or 'chamber'
36. To cut with a knife
39. In a direction toward the inion
40. A total living form
45. Has life
47. Dermato______; skin specialist
49. Metatarsus adductus
50. Mental lethargy
51. _____phoresis; ionic medication
52. _____eous; of the skin
54. ____thenar; dorsum of the hand
55. To seal or fasten with wax or cement
56. Reduces a fracture
57. ___gut; suture material
58. Human granulocytotropic ehrlichiosis (acronym)
59. Exercise-induced asthma (acronym)

31

Across

1. Rate of movement
5. Poisonous secretion of an animal
10. ____oid; lens-shaped
14. ____toid; tooth-shaped
15. _____phobia; fear of the wind
16. ____baric; below normal pressure
17. Repose after exertion
18. ______itis; inflammation of adipose tissue
19. Tip of a structure
20. Within the substance of a tonsil
23. A local astringent and styptic
24. ___iatry; study and treatment of speech disorders
25. Eyeball cavities
28. Falling out of the hair
33. ______able; soft
34. _____genic; causing sexual arousal
35. ___egumentary; relating to the skin
36. ____taxis; slight hemorrhage
37. Surgical incision (suffix)
38. ____form; resembling a vessel
39. An infusion or decoction
40. ______ment; the longitudinal position of a limb
41. The cheeks
42. Skull junction of occipital, parietal, and temporal bones
44. Stupid people
45. Symbol for microgram
46. ____uria; presence of bile pigments in the urine
47. Formation of an anuclear keratin layer
54. A mental conception
55. Laughter
56. Treat with a light beam device
57. ____itis; inflammation of the ciliary body
58. ______itis; inflammation of the innermost layer
59. ____aly; deviation from normal
60. ____gonist; agonist's opposer
61. Main artery
62. ____form; resembling a network

Down

1. Openings or foramina
2. ____algia; gland pain
3. ____algia; rib pain
4. The internal organs, especially the intestines
5. Medialis, intermedius or lateralis
6. ______ology; study of insects
7. ____cephalon; most recently evolved brain part
8. Tumors (suffix)
9. The ability to move
10. _______dynia; pain in the penis
11. ____cusis; hearing impairment
12. ____ture; an opening
13. Acronym for cyclooxygenase
21. Apparent life-threatening event (acronym)
22. _____chezia; emotional discharge gained by uttering indecent words
25. Blast_____; tumors composed of immature undifferentiated cells
26. Forces sexual intercourse
27. Tympany of the stomach or cecum
28. ______osis; a forecast of probable results
29. ____ambulism; sleepwalking
30. ______rrhea; drooling
31. ______itary; injurious to health
32. Inflammation of the sebaceous glands of the eyelids
34. ____tropic; directed against the cause
37. Abnormal indifference toward things
38. Relating to smallpox
40. Superior aortic curve
41. To shed periodically an outer covering
43. Emergency Medical Treatment and Labor Act (acronym)
44. A poisonous vapor
46. An abnormal sound heard in auscultation
47. ____acusis; painful sensitivity to noise
48. ____algia; proctalgia
49. ____cilia; motile, protoplasmic filaments on the free surface of a cell
50. ____ogen; female sex hormone
51. Of sound mind
52. ____onic; having equal tension
53. Prefix meaning 'half'
54. Islet cell antibody (acronym)

1	2	3	4			5	6	7	8	9		10	11	12
13				14		15						16		
17					18							19		
20								21			22			
			23			24	25		26					
27	28	29		30				31		32				
33				34					35		36		37	38
39			40					41		42				
43					44		45					46		
		47		48		49						50		
51	52				53		54				55			
56						57			58			59	60	61
62				63			64	65						
66				67						68				
69				70							71			

Across

1. Round, flat anatomical structure (variable)
5. Severe abdominal pain causing crying
10. ___ology; study of disease causes
13. _____itis; inflammation of the innermost layer
15. _____sis; scientific investigation
16. A metallic bone implant
17. Collapse of lung tissue
19. Spastic colon (abbrev.)
20. Prefix referring to reproductive organs
21. Normal childbirth
23. Main artery
26. One-millionth of a meter
27. Any whitish, milklike liquid
30. A unit of weight
32. Computed tomography angiography (acronym)
33. Swelling (suffix)
34. ______ation; inhalation
36. Concludes
39. Wine-cups
41. Thin slice of tissue
43. ____ordination; ataxia
44. Pertaining to a fissure
46. U.S. psychiatrists' grp.
47. ___acid; acid buffering substance
49. ______rrhea; drooling
50. ___idic; pertaining to scales
51. A wall of a body part
54. Enzyme-linked immunosorbent assay (acronym)
56. Tearlessness
58. A covering
62. ___ophobia; fear of objects to the left
63. An agent used in the treatment of burns
66. ___encephaly; occipital cranial defect, with brain exposed
67. The trunk
68. To turn outward
69. ___ophobia; fear of disease
70. Egg-shaped
71. Superior aortic curve

Down

1. ____nose; determine a disease
2. ____grity; soundness of structure
3. ____osis; a bodily passage narrowing
4. Hairlike processes projecting from cells
5. ___gut; suture material
6. ___nism; coitus interruptus
7. Treat an anatomic structure with a light beam device
8. Broad, flaring portion of the hip bone
9. Pertaining to the urinary bladder
10. Eponeurosis connecting frontalis to occipitalis
11. _____fibular; relating to the leg bones
12. _____itary; injurious to health
14. Referring to the forehead
18. A death investigator
22. Group of eight
24. A cough
25. Atrial natriuretic peptide (acronym)
27. ____thin; emulsifying phospholipid
28. Acute motor axonal neuropathy (acronym)
29. Hippocampus minor (2 words)
31. Farther from the origin
35. The state of being actual or true
37. An illicit drug
38. A short sharp sound
40. Referring to a charged particle
42. An end
45. Counterimmunoelectrophoresis (acronym)
48. ______genic; causing congenital anomalies
51. _____opsia; visual perseveration
52. _____dynia; pain in a gland
53. _____itis; joint membrane inflammation
55. Acronym for analysis of variance
57. ____phia; a wasting away
59. A tubular passage
60. ____ular; sphincteral muscle shape
61. Adrenocorticotropic hormone (acronym)
64. International sensitivity index (acronym)
65. ___algia; foot pain

1	2	3	4	■	5	6	7	8	■	9	10	11	12	13
14				■	15				■	16				
17				■	18				■	19				
20				21					22					
23						■	24				■	■	■	■
■	■	■	■	25		26		■	27		28	29	30	31
32	33	34	35		■	36		37		■	38			
39					40		■	41		42				
43				■	44		45		■	46				
47				48		■	49		50		■	■	■	■
■	■	■	■	51		52		■	53		54	55	56	57
58	59	60	61					62						
63					■	64				■	65			
66					■	67				■	68			
69					■	70				■	71			

Across

1. International Classification of Diseases (acronym)
5. Incapable of normal locomotion
9. An agreeable odor
14. Fetor ____; halitosis
15. ____tia; denoting lack of force
16. Male ejaculatory fluid
17. ____raction; act of diverting
18. Prefix meaning 'one billionth'
19. _____morphia; overall malformation
20. Within or among the epithelial cells
23. An encircling structure
24. A taste quality produced by acids
25. ____oid; ring-shaped
27. One who is affected with madness
32. _____lysis; surgical collapse of the apex of the lung
36. ____mania; hypochondriacism
38. ____mania; compulsive shopping
39. Relating to the large intestine
41. Ring-shaped
43. ____ogy; series of three
44. Set of rules, principles, or ethics
46. _____trichic; having straight hair
47. Disease-free state
49. Roman 152
51. Infraorbitomeatal line (acronym)
53. The inherent character of life
58. ________________ accident; stroke
63. _____osis; incomplete development of the body
64. ____ment; bone-connecting tissue
65. A unit of perceived loudness
66. Line
67. ____cephalon; thalamus and hypothalamus
68. ____oid; S-shaped
69. Larynx sound
70. Midway between front and back
71. ____phobia; fear of different mental conceptions

Down

1. Relating to iodine
2. _____genic; causing secretion
3. _____action; act of diverting
4. _____cyte; star-shaped cell
5. Straight
6. Anionic neutrophil-activating peptide (acronym)
7. _______cyte; sickle cell
8. _____genic; causing sexual arousal
9. Rough
10. Having verifiable existence
11. Prefix meaning 'universally'
12. prefix meaning 'beyond' or 'after'
13. ____eptic; nervous system stimulant
21. Elbow
22. A body fluid, such as blood, lymph, or bile
26. ____ordination; ataxia
28. ____ceptor; free nerve ending that detects pain
29. ____emia; excess fibrin in the blood
30. Sup. rectus femoris attachment pt.
31. ____genic; formed by a genetic sequence
32. Adrenocorticotropic hormone (acronym)
33. Minute opening of the skin
34. ____cus; hip flexor
35. ____iculus; small mound
37. ____algia; leg pain
40. A thin serous discharge from a wound
42. _____ crest; pelvic ridge
45. Roman 658
48. Shin bones
50. Of unsound mind
52. Various microscopic fungi
54. _____genic; causing cough
55. Resembling a scar
56. The difference between the limits of a variable
57. _____phobia; fear of solitude
58. ____arium; braincase portion of the skull
59. ____tropic; directed against the cause
60. ____capsule; capsule of the kidney
61. ____tive; not essential
62. Old

1	2	3	4	5	■	6	7	8	■	9	10	11	12	13
14					■	15			■	16				
17					■	18			19					
20					■	21						■	■	■
■	■	22			■	23				■	24	25	26	27
28	29			■	30				■	■	31			
32			■	33				■	34	35				
36			37				■	38						
39						■	40				■	41		
42				■	■	43				■	44			
45				■	46				■	47			■	■
■	■	■	48	49					■	50			51	52
53	54	55							■	56				
57					■	58			■	59				
60					■	61			■	62				

Across

1. The line of union of the halves of various symmetrical parts
6. ___cine; resistance-builder
9. Dorsal
14. _____ology; study of dreams
15. ___tropic; influencing muscular contractility
16. Speak one`s mind
17. Prefix referring to the ankle
18. Inflammation of the eyeball's outer layer
20. Expectorates
21. A cylindrical anatomic part
22. Counterimmunoelectrophoresis (acronym)
23. ____esis; involuntary discharge of urine
24. Infection-associated hemophagocytic syndrome (acronym)
28. ____genesis; reproduction by segmentation
30. Metric unit of weight
31. ____roid; resembling a dream
32. Wing-like process
33. Alumnus
34. A group of five
36. Monthly
38. Submissive
39. Any equal part
40. ____ated; charged with iron
41. ___ anum; 'through the anus'
42. Acute motor axonal neuropathy (acronym)
43. Prefix meaning 'large intestine'
44. ____philia; pathological interest in filth
45. ____atry; study and treatment of speech disorders
46. ____gate; to wash out
47. ___epinephrine; a vasoconstrictor
48. Fine, soft, lightly pigmented fetal hair
50. _____osis; incomplete development of the body
53. Inflammation of the lip
56. Laughter
57. Ate_____sis; collapse of lung tissue
58. Roman 106
59. _____phobia; fear of sexual intercourse
60. _____ia; silver poisoning
61. Hydroxyethyl starch (acronym)
62. Beginning

Down

1. Decays
2. Anionic neutrophil-activating peptide (acronym)
3. Surrounding the skull
4. Prefix meaning 'tissue'
5. Irregularly notched, toothed, or indented
6. Pertaining to an internal organ
7. Toward the elbow
8. The neck
9. The average
10. Subjective beliefs
11. Female breast (slang)
12. ___lingus; sexual stimulation of the anus
13. ___bian; female homosexual
19. An___ysm; blood vessel bulge
25. The state of being free from fever
26. Retches
27. ______penia; iron deficiency
28. Vertebrate that possesses hair and suckle their young
29. Oil tumor
30. CNS 'matter' consisting of nonmyelinated nerve tissue
33. The intestine or stomach
34. ____dynia; labor pains
35. Erythrocyte sedimentation rate (acronym)
37. Loss of mental abilities due to old age
38. ________ hepatis; a mottled blue liver
40. Pardon or excuse
43. Body weight supporting device
44. Process of changing position
46. ___encephaly; occipital cranial defect, with brain exposed
47. _____lepsy; excessive sleep disorder
49. Like a wing
51. To seal or fasten with wax or cement
52. ____onic; having equal tension
53. Clinical Laboratory Assistant (acronym)
54. She
55. Electrocardiogram (acronym)

1	2	3	4	■	5	6	7	8	■	9	10	11	12	13
14				■	15				■	16				
17				■	18				■	19				
20				21					22				■	■
23			■	24			■	■	25				26	27
28			29		■	■	30	31			■	32		
■	■	■	33		34	35				■	36			
■	■	37								38			■	■
39	40			■	41							■	■	■
42			■	43				■	■	44		45	46	47
48			49			■	■	50	51		■	52		
■	■	53				54	55				56			
57	58				■	59				■	60			
61					■	62				■	63			
64					■	65				■	66			

Across

1. ____men; earwax
5. Calcium pyrophosphate deposition disease (acronym)
9. _____osis; bone mass within a bone
14. ____toe; hallux varus
15. Winglike structures
16. Dura _____; outer brain and spinal cord membrane
17. Specific sites
18. ____osis; state of stupor
19. _____genic; causing sexual arousal
20. Enlargement of limb or genetalia
23. Cardiovascular system (acronym)
24. Alanine aminotransferase (acronym)
25. Female sibling
28. An eggshell
30. Short sleeps
32. Exercise-induced asthma (acronym)
33. _______meter; caliper used to measure the size of testes
36. Hairless
37. Within the ankle
39. ____section; phlebotomy
41. Not containing a liquid
42. Intramuscular stimulation (acronym)
43. ____nal; everlasting
44. 1st letter of the Greek alphabet
48. Lying face up
50. Roman 650
52. Petroleum
53. Within the cerebrum
57. _____megaly; enlargement of an atrium
59. ____centesis; surgical puncture of the large intestine
60. 9th letter in the Greek alphabet
61. Sleep image
62. Rainbow-like eye part
63. Acute motor axonal neuropathy (acronym)
64. ______pathy; intervertebral cartilage disease
65. ____algia; pain in the back
66. Sodium chloride

Down

1. ______asia; distention of the large intestine
2. Develop
3. A small hollow
4. ____osia; drinking of urine
5. A narrow passage
6. _____algia; pain in the sole of the foot
7. A portion
8. Prefix indicating 'one tenth'
9. Vomiting
10. Nostril
11. Relating to the ossicles of the ear
12. To reduce a fracture
13. ___chanter; bony elevation
21. Highly active antiretroviral therapy (acronym)
22. ______genous; not producing spores
26. ___oid; resembling a coil or roll
27. A unit of energy absorbed from ionizing radiation
29. A sound of distinct frequency
30. Saltpeter
31. Adenosine deaminase acting on RNA (acronym)
34. The most depressed central portion of an ulcer
35. Hereditary angioneurotic edema (acronym)
36. Basic activities of daily living (acronym)
37. Inhales
38. _____mesis; vomiting of saliva
39. Force, energy, or power
40. Medicinal Australian bird oil
43. ______phobia; fear of insects
45. Benign tumor lining the skin openings of sweat glands
46. Referring to an opening
47. ______oid; sausage-shaped
49. Relating to the inion
50. _____ious; affected by acute confusion
51. _____-eye; esotropia
54. Ascorbic ____; vitamin C
55. ____meter; pupillometer
56. A prejudiced or subjective attitude
57. ___uction; movement toward midline
58. Prefix meaning 'three'

Across

1. _____genic; causing disease
6. A short sharp sound
10. ____ralopia; day blindness
14. Follows orders
15. Bridge between medulla and midbrain
16. ____emia; blood volume deficiency
17. _____ole; heart relaxation phase
18. Prefix meaning 'eight'
19. Insect parasite that causes scabies
20. Separation of two adjacent bones
23. ____phobia; fear of the dawn
24. _____osis; degeneration of collagen fibers
25. Gains knowledge through experience
28. _____phobia; fear of speaking or stuttering
31. ____gate; to wash out
32. Referring to a charged particle
33. Diagnostic and Statistical Manual of Mental Disorders (abbrev.)
36. Absence of the cerebellum
40. International sensitivity index (acronym)
41. Relating to the inion
42. Brittle hair, impaired intelligence, decreased fertility, and short stature (abbrev.)
43. Evacuated fecal matter
44. A wall of a body part
46. _____genation; interbreeding of different races
49. ____tectomy; removal of the liver
50. Narrowing of the intestinal lumen
56. ____osis; a bodily passage narrowing
57. Having verifiable existence
58. Digital Imaging and Communications in Medicine (abbrev.)
60. ____algia; main artery pain
61. Roman 152
62. Relating to iodine
63. A toothlike structure
64. A luminous circle
65. _____esia; pain insensibility

Down

1. ___algia; foot pain
2. ____genesis; development of life from nonlife
3. Decoctions
4. Excessive or uncontrollable emotion
5. Basic unit of structure of compact bone
6. _____genous; caused by waste material
7. ____ceptor; free nerve ending that detects pain
8. ____gonist; agonist's opposer
9. Upper attachment point for posterior sacroiliac ligament (abbrev.)
10. ______cephalus; having a flattened head
11. Enzyme-linked immunosorbent assay (acronym)
12. Mild
13. To discharge waste
21. ___iferous; producing bone
22. _____opsia; migraine aura
25. ____ment; liquid preparation rubbed into the skin
26. The sum of all instincts for self-preservation
27. ____culus; joint
28. Not general or systemic
29. ____dotal; based on case histories
30. Labium
32. ____pagus; twins joined at the occiput
33. Roman 552
34. Midway between front and back
35. A quantity of matter
37. Saltpeter
38. ___phthalmos; recession of the eyeball
39. Surface scraping
43. Odors
44. ___ectomy; surgical removal of the penis
45. Absence of feet
46. Toward the median plane of the body
47. Metatarsus adductus
48. _____algia; breastbone pain
49. _____phobia; fear of the sun
51. ____itis; inflammation of the testis
52. ____phobia; fear of light flashes
53. Cauda
54. International Classification of Diseases (acronym)
55. Dirt
59. Symbol for microgram

37

Across

1. Roman 801
6. ____dotal; based on case histories
10. ____naceous; soapy
14. Gain knowledge through experience
15. The cheek
16. Anionic neutrophil-activating peptide (acronym)
17. Unreasonable
19. ____algia; tooth pain
20. ___rology; the science of medicine
21. A single
22. _______glossia; congenital fissure of the tongue
24. A baby's bed
25. Habitual spasmodic muscular movements
26. Pertaining to balance and hearing
31. Genetic functional unit controlling production of a messenger RNA
32. ___unogen; antigen
33. Experimental study place
35. Lesser
36. Iminodiacetate (acronym)
37. Protective coverings on the dorsal distal phalanges
39. ___acid; acid buffering substance
40. ___nism; coitus interruptus
41. Pimple-like formation
42. Giant cell tumor of bone
46. _____phagia; ingestion of an excessive quantity of salts
47. A thickening of the skin on the toe
48. Hydroperitoneum
51. Human monocytotropic ehrlichiosis (acronym)
52. Multiple epiphysial dysplasia (acronym)
55. ____ugator; wrinkle-producing muscle
56. Abnormal smallness of one or more extremities
59. Opening at the end of the digestive system
60. ____plegia; paralysis of one limb
61. A standard of perfection
62. ____algia; proctalgia
63. A looplike structure
64. _____mention; reproduction by germination

Down

1. Roman 552
2. Wax
3. ____ilage; joint covering
4. ___vat; a type of cloth bandage
5. Medial rotator
6. Single-celled organism (variable)
7. ___ism; dwarfishness
8. Tumorlike deposit of elastic tissue
9. Chemical found in body tissues, especially bone
10. One who delights in cruelty
11. ____thesia; lack of sensation
12. To breathe rapidly and shallowly
13. ___kinetic; pertaining to eye movement
18. The most prominent craniometric point at the occipital protuberance
23. Human chorionic somatomammotropic hormone (abbrev.)
24. ____tid; neck artery
26. _____cellular; pertaining to prickle cells
27. Bed coverings for administering oxygen
28. Suffix meaning 'killing'
29. Broad, flaring portion of the hip bone
30. Common acute lymphoblastic leukemia antigen (acronym)
31. Tumor (suffix)
34. Abbreviation for breast self-examination
36. The act of cutting
37. Presence of sodium in the blood
38. ____eurosis; sheet-like tendon
40. Plasma membrane of the oocyte
41. _____phagia; swallowing food without thorough mastication
43. A desire to drink
44. Consume
45. ______cyte; a colorless cell
48. ____ology; study of mites and ticks
49. A unit of perceived loudness
50. _____iate; cross-shaped
52. ____tive; not essential
53. ____rhea; liquid feces
54. Masculine
57. Brain and spinal cord system (abbrev.)
58. Expected date of confinement (acronym)

38

Across

1. A quantity of matter
5. Chronic progressive external ophthalmoplegia (acronym)
9. ____locephalus; having a flattened head
13. Short for 'death notice'
14. Ate_____sis; collapse of lung tissue
16. ____aly; deviation from normal
17. Refuse to admit
18. Muscle protein localized in the I band of myofibrils
19. Prefix signifying one quadrillion
20. To emerge through
22. The state produced by fulfillment of a specific need
24. Smallest unit of an element
26. Rounded, flat plates
27. Pertaining to vision
30. A scroll-like bone found in the skull
33. Causing an increase of flesh
35. _____esthesia; phantom limb pain
37. ___lingus; sexual stimulation of the anus
38. Inwardly
41. Roman 1600
42. Pierces with a pointed instrument
45. Echo-free
48. Lipogranuloma
51. A gas under pressure
52. _____omosis; blood vessel coalescence
54. Prefix meaning 'after'
55. Excludes unconsciously from the conscious mind
59. A delimited area
62. Toward the mouth
63. _____ology; scientific knowledge
65. ____onic; having equal tension
66. To eye provocatively
67. Small openings into hollow organs
68. Motion picture
69. A ridge formed by the doubling back of a lamina
70. ____atrial node; pacemaker
71. ____ogen; female sex hormone

Down

1. A particular condition of functioning
2. ____rant; deviating
3. __________ node; cardiac pacemaker
4. Having an astringent or hemostatic effect
5. Clinical Laboratory Assistant (acronym)
6. Short for chest muscles
7. Outward
8. Pertaining to ear inflammation
9. The science of touch
10. ____roid; resembling a dream
11. ____facient; causing movement
12. Acute motor axonal neuropathy (acronym)
15. _____coria; asymmetric pupils
21. ____phobia; fear of childbirth
23. American College of Nuclear Physicians (acronym)
25. Spouse
27. Obstructive sleep apnea syndrome (acronym)
28. _____gamy; sexual promiscuousness
29. ___itis; inflammation of gastric cellular tissue
31. The stoppage of bleeding
32. _____genic; caused by sound
34. Computed tomography angiography (acronym)
36. Roman 750
39. ___biosis; resuscitation
40. Away from the surface
43. Having facial hair
44. A unit of perceived loudness
46. Contralateral routing of signal (acronym)
47. Institution providing palliative care and support to dying people and their families
49. _____dynia; breast pain
50. Evaluate
53. _____form; roof-shaped
55. Upper surface of an anatomical structure
56. Prefix meaning 'work'
57. ____esthesia; perception of vibration
58. Anterior border of tibia
60. ____agious; communicable
61. ____nal; everlasting
64. ___pathia; seasickness

39

Across

1. Away from the surface
5. A population of identical cells
10. Adenosine 5-phosphosulfate (abbrev.)
13. ____esis; suppression of a discharge
14. Material which condoms are made from
15. Walking unit
16. Without a mouth
18. Organisms basic structural and functional unit
19. Carrier of genetic information (abbrev.)
20. Return to the normal
22. State of being joined by bone formation
26. Coatomer protein (acronym)
27. Prefix relating to the main ankle bone
28. ___chanter; bony elevation
29. 23rd letter of the Greek alphabet
30. Actual juice of the poppy
32. Roman 952
36. Smallest unit of an element
38. Bubbling sounds in the lungs
40. Acute inflammatory demyelinating polyradiculoneuropathy (acronym)
41. Sudden overpowering fright
43. Common acute lymphoblastic leukemia antigen (acronym)
45. A decoction
46. Congestive heart failure (acronym)
48. Ratio of output to input of an amplifying system
49. ___hazard; lacking any coherent system
50. Surgical puncture of an ovary
55. _______algia; painful menstrual cramps
56. Computed tomography angiography (acronym)
57. ____olic; growth enhancing steroid
58. Between the epiphysis and diaphysis
64. A measure of duration
65. A vivid mental picture
66. Soft inner substance of a hair
67. ___ulus; ringlike structure
68. ____trum; initial breast fluid
69. To catch sight of

Down

1. ___phragm; breathing muscle
2. Suffix referring to the female
3. Eversion of the eyelid edge
4. _____phobia; fear of one's own voice
5. Clinical Laboratory Assistant (acronym)
6. Short for arm adductor
7. ___dynia; earache
8. _____tis; inflammation of a nerve
9. To excise
10. _____osis; incomplete development of the body
11. _____spondylitis; inflammation of pelvic portion of spine
12. _____ectopia; floating spleen
15. Blind spot within the visual field
17. _____dynia; breast pain
21. ____ology; anatomy of the soft parts of the body
22. A rib
23. ____ophagous; feeding on decaying matter
24. _____ crest; pelvic ridge
25. Kneading and pressure of the muscles
26. Continuous positive airway pressure (acronym)
31. _____cholia; a mental depression
33. The formation of gall or kidney stones
34. Mental conceptions
35. Inspiratory positive airway pressure (acronym)
37. A very tiny form of life
39. A long, narrow opening
42. ____algia; hand pain
44. _____oic; echo-free
47. Relating to ants
50. Tumors (suffix)
51. Any poisonous substance found in snake venom
52. _____esis; recollection
53. _____therapy; drug treatment for cancer
54. A tampon
59. ___algia; ankle pain
60. Gone by
61. Foot
62. Inosine triphosphate (acronym)
63. Timid

1	2	3	4	■	5	6	7	8	9	■	10	11	12	13
14				■	15					■	16			
17				■	18					■	19			
20				21						22	■	23		
24					■	■	25				■	26		
27			■	28	29	30	■	■	31		32			
■	■	■	33				34	35	■	■	36			
■	■	37							38	39			■	■
40	41			■	■	42						■	■	■
43				44	45	■	■	46			■	47	48	49
50			■	51		52	53	■	■	54	55			
56			■	57				58	59					
60			61	■	62					■	63			
64				■	65					■	66			
67				■	68					■	69			

Across

1. Tumors (suffix)
5. Knocks senseless
10. ____tus; the motor element of an instinct
14. ____cardia; enlargement of the heart
15. _____phobia; fear of poverty
16. Inert gaseous element in the atmosphere
17. ____uria; extravasation of urine
18. _____ment; longitudinal position of a limb
19. ____ectomy; surgical removal of part of the iris
20. Defective development of one side of the mandible
23. Obstructive sleep apnea (acronym)
24. Negatively charged ion
25. ____osis; a bodily passage narrowing
26. Prefix meaning 'seed' or 'semen'
27. Whitish, milklike liquid
28. Nonlymphoid blood cancer (abbrev.)
31. Physically powerful
33. ______form; resembling a goiter
36. ____form; loop-shaped
37. Science of speech disorders
40. ____phobia; fear of childbirth
42. Element/mineral used in the synthesis of thyroid hormones
43. Decayed
46. Organic mood syndrome (acronym)
47. ___bian; female homosexual
50. International Prognostic Index (acronym)
51. ____phase; final stage of mitosis or meiosis
54. _____ation; belching
56. Roman 155
57. Lack of desire or craving
60. Pilus
62. _____itis; inflammation of the innermost layer
63. Pre-migraine sensation
64. ____mus; narrow passage between two parts
65. Alveoli
66. ____oris; erectile female organ
67. ____esthesia; absence of muscle sensation
68. ate_____sis; collapse of lung tissue
69. ____dynia; sinew pain

Down

1. ______itis; inflammation of umbilicus
2. Passage of dark-colored, tarry stools
3. Reproducing without the union of male and female cells
4. _____purulent; characterized by bloody pus
5. The full extent of anything
6. Any weblike tissue
7. Components of a whole
8. _____mare; horrible dream
9. Thin, blood-stained, purulent discharge
10. ___encephaly; occipital cranial defect, with brain exposed
11. Incomplete development of an ovum
12. Substances injurious to health
13. _______itis; inflammation of the intima of a blood vessel
21. _____ology; study of the masticatory apparatus
22. ___acid; acid buffering substance
29. Blood flow imaging technique (abbrev.)
30. ____tropy; myocardial relaxation
32. Violent anger
33. Macula
34. Prefix meaning 'less'
35. ____therapy; treatment with iodine
37. Presence of neurogenic electrical energy
38. ___bus; border or margin
39. Beginning
40. Glosso_______; hairy tongue
41. Protoplasmic portion of the ovum
44. ___ology; study of disease causes
45. Refusal to admit reality
47. A small semilunar structure
48. ______ology; study of exocrine glands
49. ______lysis; fat emulsion in the digestive process
52. To incise with a sharp object
53. Pertaining to sight
55. Respond to a stimulus
58. 16 fluid ounces (U.S.)
59. Condition of blood (suffix)
61. 17th letter of the Greek alphabet

Across

1. ____nestic; assisting the memory
5. Control of Communicable Diseases Manual (acronym)
9. _____nant; cancerous
14. ____dynia; sinew pain
15. Chief nitrogenous endproduct of protein metabolism
16. Anal injection of fluid
17. To restore to health
18. ____atomic; denoting five atoms per molecule
19. Normal firmness in body tissues
20. Narrowing of the intestinal lumen
23. A system of extreme religious beliefs and rituals
24. ___didymus; single body conjoined twins
25. goiter
28. ____formis; external hip rotator
30. Arteriovenous anastomosis (acronym)
33. To remove the outer layer by stripping
34. Injures
35. ___centric; having a common center
36. Between the neuromeres
40. Roman 52
41. _____power; unit of power
42. Prefix meaning 'one trillionth'
43. ___ugo; fine fetal body hair
44. Critical stage of a disease
45. ______head; quality of being a virgin
47. Cognitive-behavioral therapy (acronym)
48. The fat of swine
49. Referring to the heart and blood vessels
56. _____stasis; state of equilibrium
57. ____algia; proctalgia
58. Nerve branches
59. _____ferous; Conveying urine
60. ____ordination; ataxia
61. Acrocephalosyndactyly (abbrev.)
62. Inwardly
63. Dread
64. ____emia; white blood cell disease

Down

1. ____roma; artery wall mass
2. ____cephalon; most recently evolved brain part
3. ____omy; body structure study
4. Smallest unit of a substance
5. Dome-shaped cap
6. Bone ridge
7. ____algia; tooth pain
8. Spouse
9. Persistence of the frontal suture in the adult
10. _____gnosia; denial of a neurological deficit
11. ____tive; a demulcent remedy
12. Most inferior of several similar structures
13. Flatulence
21. Spirit distilled from sugar cane
22. _____cyte; healthy red blood cell
25. Overflow
26. Any anatomic, bandlike structure
27. _____itis; inflammation of the optomeninx
28. Temporary stop
29. ____versible; permanent
30. Unpleasant to the smell or taste
31. Larynx sound
32. Elbow
34. ____aphrodite; intersexual person
37. Rod-shaped
38. _____phobia; morbid dread of night
39. External to dura mater
45. ______rhagia; hemorrhage from a breast
46. AIDS-related complex (abbrev.)
47. A V-shaped cut
48. Shellac
49. A thickening of the skin on the toe
50. ____osis; direct nuclear division
51. Open reduction and internal fixation (acronym)
52. ____section; phlebotomy
53. ____rated; torn
54. ____tate; cut off
55. Possible peril of a treatment
56. A shade or tint

42

Across

1. Vertical in position
6. Any of various parasitic insects
11. International Prognostic Index (acronym)
14. A water-soluble carbohydrate
15. Incus
16. ___tropics; brain enhancers
17. Within bone
19. Stannum
20. Resistant to change
21. Something that nourishes
23. ___dynia; earache
24. ______gnathia; open bite
25. ____eurosis; sheet-like tendon
28. One-hundredth of a right angle
32. VD
33. ___emia; dissolution of red blood cells
34. _____liptics; treatment by inunction
36. A cleft or crack
39. Proximal upper limb parts
41. The rate of change of position with time
42. Grows older
43. Lowermost attaching structure
44. Weblike tissues
45. Intrinsic sympathomimetic activity (acronym)
46. ___cyx; tailbone
48. _____ambulism; sleepwalking
49. Smallest unit of an element
50. Small cavity within a tissue
53. ___ology; study of tumors
55. An exact copy
57. Congenital absence of the spinal cord
61. Glucose tolerance test (acronym)
62. Any professional misconduct
64. ___facial; relating to the mouth and face
65. An abnormal sound heard in auscultation
66. Neoplasm
67. ___epinephrine; a vasoconstrictor
68. ______loquy; sleeptalking
69. ______phobia; fear of rain

Down

1. Condition, action, or process (suffix)
2. The smallest of a litter
3. Ethyleneglycotetraacetic acid (acronym)
4. The most widely distributed element
5. A qualitative characteristic
6. Treat with a light beam device
7. ___ology; metaphysical study of the nature of being and existence
8. Pigmented vascular layer of the eyeball
9. _____denitis; salivary gland inflammation
10. ______oid; oval-shaped
11. The area of the hand or foot lying between adjacent digits
12. A sharp end or apex
13. ______phoresis; ionic medication
18. Specialist (suffix)
22. Uterus
25. Like a wing
26. ____genic; producing fever
27. A receptor in the anterior hypothalamus that responds to osmotic pressure
29. Forces sexual intercourse
30. Prefix meaning 'imperfect or incomplete'
31. Sleep image
35. Benign epithelial neoplasm with a basic glandular structure
37. ____morph; large, strong body type
38. Acute sensory axonal motor neuropathy (abbrev.)
40. Evacuated fecal matter
47. Ascends
49. Vinegar
50. A colorless, odorless gas; atomic no. 18
51. _____grade; moving backward
52. _____phobia; fear of small skin parasites
54. _____philia; preference for the night
56. A local astringent and styptic
57. ____culus; joint
58. An arm or leg
59. ____rhea; maintenance of water equilibrium
60. ____genesis; the formation of gas
63. A metallic bone implant

43

Across

1. The body of a nerve cell
5. ____tern; reservoir
9. _____itis; penis head inflammation
14. Progesterone (acronym)
15. Pilus
16. _____genic; starch-forming
17. Prefix meaning 'work'
18. ____genous; native to
19. _____thropy; delusion that one is a wolf
20. Brain part concerned with smell
23. Large, back chewing tooth
24. Narrow elevation of a bone
25. Gain knowledge through experience
29. ______ bile duct; duct that empties bile into the duodenum
33. Director of Medical Education (acronym)
36. A blood clot
38. International Classification of Diseases (acronym)
39. Cerebral hemorrhage
43. Material from which the glaze for artificial teeth is made
44. To look fixedly
45. ___tropic; influencing muscular contractility
46. Decayed
49. Relating to the distal small intestinal section
51. ____cent; free from wrong
53. Larynx sound
57. In front and to the inner side
62. Terminal portion of the small intestine
63. Dys____; difficulty in breathing
64. Diethylenetriamine pentaacetic acid (acronym)
65. _____ equina; distal end of the spinal cord
66. ____ital; health care institution
67. Rainbow-like eye part
68. _____ major; arm adductor
69. ____itis; inflammation of a bone
70. Sodium chloride

Down

1. Male reproductive cell
2. _____diagnosis; serum diagnosis
3. _____alia; pathological speech problem
4. Pertaining to painful death
5. The mentum
6. International Anatomical Nomenclature Committee (acronym)
7. Midway between front and back
8. _____opia; perception of three images of an object
9. ______plasty; surgical repair of the glans penis
10. Excess starch in the blood
11. ____pene; red pigment of a tomato
12. ____ine; an amino acid
13. ___cellular; lacking cellular organization
21. Vertical in position
22. ___cup; diaphragmatic spasm
26. ___flexia; lack of reflexes
27. Moves swiftly on foot
28. _____phobia; morbid dread of night
30. Roman 1151
31. ____toid; tooth-shaped
32. Prefix meaning 'one billionth'
33. Dihydrofolate reductase (acronym)
34. ____genesis; reproduction by segmentation
35. Enzyme-multiplied immunoassay technique (acronym)
37. Having verifiable existence
40. Position of the body and limbs
41. Prefix meaning 'before'
42. Retch
47. Anal injections of fluid
48. Abbreviation for 'do not resuscitate'
50. Of the heart
52. _____rrhagia; ovarian hemorrhage
54. Prefix meaning 'within'
55. _____lary; microscopic blood vessel
56. _____osis; degeneration of collagen fibers
57. Winglike structures
58. ____algia; nerve pain
59. ____emia; excess fibrin in the blood
60. A small mass of foreign cells
61. Synthetic material used as a suture
62. ___erus; jaundice

Across

1. Roman 1106
5. _____ cranial nerve; olfactory
10. ____ular; sphincteral muscle shape
14. ____itis; inflammation of the elbow joint
15. _____noid; weblike
16. ____algia; gland pain
17. A shade of a color
18. Saltpeter
19. Prefix meaning 'digestion'
20. Within the adenoids
23. Pertaining to minute, infectious agents
24. Abbreviation for Epstein-Barr virus
25. To elicit a tendon reflex
27. Prefix meaning 'habitat'
28. A local astringent and styptic
32. Lying face up
34. A type of cloth bandage
36. Decays
37. Removal of spots or other blemishes from the skin
40. Prefix meaning 'all' or 'everywhere'
42. Fats that are insoluble in water
43. Moving
46. Biological unit of heredity
47. U.S. hospital gp.
50. ___dontia; absence of teeth
51. Inosine triphosphate (acronym)
53. _____oid; resembling a star
55. Examination of the interior of the eye
60. _____genous; originating outside the organism
61. In a direction toward the inion
62. _____omy; body structure study
63. ____psoas; hip flexor
64. ______geal; of the tailbone
65. Seizure made with the teeth
66. Head and trunk connector
67. _____algia; breastbone pain
68. To examine with a sensing device

Down

1. Learned drive
2. A treatment facility
3. ________lateral; to the front and the side
4. Prefix meaning 'within'
5. Abbreviation for fluorescent antinuclear antibody test
6. ____ectomy; surgical removal of part of the iris
7. Frequency that an event occurs per unit of time
8. Exhibition of questionable behavior
9. Pulsates
10. Continuous ambulatory peritoneal dialysis (acronym)
11. The formation of conceptions
12. Surgically reattach a body part to the original site
13. Brain and spinal cord system (abbrev.)
21. 'As low as reasonably achievable' (acronym)
22. Intravenous urogram (acronym)
26. Foot
29. Any whitish, milklike liquid
30. ____optosis; staphylodialysis
31. ______nant; cancerous
33. ____encephalon; forebrain
34. Roman 902
35. Synthetic material used as a suture
37. Within the eyeball
38. Stannum
39. Mental conceptions
40. Tumor (suffix)
41. A single ophthalmic lens
44. ___mus; acidity or alkalinity indicator
45. Values and guidelines
47. Lacking normal muscle tone
48. _______trophia; liver atrophy
49. _______oid; pitcher-shaped
52. ______itis; inflammation of the entire ear
54. Crusts of superficial sores
56. Hamulus
57. Small, flat-bodied, wingless biting or sucking insects
58. ____ocyte; large red blood cell
59. ____acusis; painful sensitivity to noise
60. Endometrial intraepithelial neoplasia (acronym)

45

Across

1. Hexamethyl-propyleneamine oxime (acronym)
6. Any weblike tissue
10. Prefix meaning 'within'
14. The time during which someone's life continues
15. Expiratory positive airway pressure (acronym)
16. ____opsy; autopsy
17. Portions
18. Narrow elevation of a bone
19. Roman 800
20. Agent that prevents or arrests vomiting
22. ____itis; inflammation of the testis
23. Interstitial cell-stimulating hormone (acronym)
24. Blood clots circulating in the blood
26. ____pathic; of unknown origin
30. ___ pack; cold local application
31. Roman 601
32. ____hosis; liver disorder
33. 9th letter in the Greek alphabet
35. A rib
39. A congenital defect in the upper lip
41. The act of touching
43. _____genic; appetite stimulating
44. ____genous; originating outside the organism
46. A mental conception
47. ___antile; denoting childish behavior
49. She
50. Protective plaster shell
51. Dys______; difficulty in swallowing
54. ____geny; development of an organism
56. A network of nerves or blood vessels
57. Communicable by contact
63. Not obstructed
64. ____genous; native to
65. _____genesis; milk production
66. ____pedic; clubfooted
67. ____phobia; fear of heights
68. _____algia; intestinal pain
69. Aural
70. Lumbus
71. Numerical evaluation of achievement

Down

1. ____cusis; hearing impairment
2. An average
3. A portion
4. ____culus; joint
5. Inter_____ dorsales; hand muscles
6. Optic instrument used to visualize distant objects
7. Characterizing term or name
8. ____ary; adapted for tearing
9. Autoimmune polyendocrinopathy-candidiasis-ectodermal dystrophy (acronym)
10. Living as a parasite within the host
11. _____phobia; fear of dying
12. Roman 850
13. _____algia; pain in the testes
21. Roman 1103
25. Roman 1300
26. ____roid; denoting a thin purulent discharge
27. ____rhea; liquid feces
28. ____versible; permanent
29. Appetite stimulating
34. The ability to focus
36. French for AIDS
37. Foot digits
38. ____omy; body structure study
40. ____ment; liquid preparation rubbed into the skin
42. Main artery
45. _______fication; cartilage formation
48. Pertaining to front of the head
51. _____plast; one that is formed first
52. _____itis; inflammation of the liver
53. _____osis; incomplete development of the body
55. Eyes provocatively
58. _____genesis; origin and growth of a neoplasm
59. International Anatomical Nomenclature Committee (acronym)
60. Prefix meaning 'eight'
61. ____itis; inflammation in the womb
62. Tender

46

Across

1. ____roid; denoting a thin purulent discharge

5. Crusts of superficial sores

10. ____phobia; fear of marriage

14. Foot digits

15. _____plasty; pupil procedure

16. Like a wing

17. ____oid; ring-shaped

18. _____ferous; yielding milk

19. ____ually; toward the tongue

20. Unilateral headache

23. _____pelvis; twisted pelvis

24. Occurring on the 9th day

25. ______lysis; fat emulsion in the digestive process

28. ____ose; fatty

30. Warmth

31. Poisonous secretion of an animal

33. Arterial blood gas (acronym)

36. Between the metatarsal bones

40. ___ophobia; fear of disease

41. Pertaining to a stroke or seizure

42. ____form; shaped like a leather bottle

43. Ova

44. The early stage of a developing organism

46. _____genous; of ligamentous origin

49. A person with Hansen disease

51. Between the collarbones

57. A sitting surface

58. The extremities of any axis

59. Violent anger

60. Roman 902

61. Alveoli

62. ____onic; having equal tension

63. International Anatomical Nomenclature Committee (acronym)

64. _____receptor; detects light

65. ____bellum; movement coordinator

Down

1. Scratch trigger

2. The central part of a structure

3. ____lich; abdominal thrust maneuver

4. To yawn

5. Prefix meaning 'hard'

6. To join together

7. _____cerebellum: oldest part (variable)

8. Cells that produce insulin

9. Dirt

10. A triple cadence to the heart sounds

11. _____ment; the longitudinal position of a limb

12. Madness

13. Body structure with a specific function

21. A small collapsible bed

22. The soul or life

25. Anterior border of tibia

26. ____dynia; sinew pain

27. Consumes

28. ____eptic; nervous system stimulant

29. Directly observed therapy (acronym)

31. Pet docs

32. 7th letter of the Greek alphabet

33. ____oid; star-shaped

34. ____phonia; thick, heavy voice quality

35. ____blast; early neural cell

37. _____ mortis; death state

38. Symbol for microgram

39. Pertaining to reddish urine

43. An agent that induces vomitting

44. ______plasty; plastic surgery of the vulva

45. ___ism; abnormal prolongation of part of the body

46. Rounded, flat plates

47. Anal injection of fluid

48. To dye

49. _____phobia; fear of speaking or stuttering

50. Specific occurrence

52. Continuous positive airway pressure (acronym)

53. ____iorrhea; excessive, post-childbirth, vaginal discharge

54. Treat with a light beam device

55. ____aphobia; fear of public places

56. An anatomical network

■	■	1	2	3	■	4	5	6	7	■	8	9	10	11
■	12				■	13				■	14			
15					■	16				17				
18					19				■	20				
21			■	22			■	■	23					
24			25			■	26	27			■	28		
29					■	30				■	31			
■	■	■	32		33					34		■	■	■
35	36	37		■	38				■	39		40	41	42
43			■	44				■	45					
46			47			■	■	48			■	49		
50					■	51	52				53			
54					55				■	56				
57				■	58				■	59				■
60				■	61				■	62			■	■

Across

1. Abbreviation for epithelial membrane antigen

4. Abbreviation for other licensed antifungal therapies

8. Part of a surface

12. The sum of all instincts for self-preservation

13. ____ocyte; large red blood cell

14. ____ugator; wrinkle-producing muscle

15. To put forth effort

16. Instrument for evacuating fluid or tissue by suction

18. Causes an inclination to vomit

20. A salt of uric acid

21. ___ology; metaphysical study of the nature of being and existence

22. Carrier of genetic information (abbrev.)

23. Inflammation of fibrous tissue

24. ______metry; measurement of muscular strength

26. ____ose; milk sugar

28. ___ectomy; excision of a bone

29. ______centesis; puncture and drainage of the thoracic cavity

30. Abbreviation for fetal alcohol spectrum disorders

31. Proximal upper limb parts

32. An early neural cell

35. ____dysphoria; abnormal dislike of certain odors

38. A long, narrow opening

39. Pace

43. Abbreviation for chimpanzee coryza agent

44. ____dynia; foot pain

45. Pertaining to the abdomen

46. A suture material

48. ___cellular; lacking cellular organization

49. ___iculation; joint

50. Pertaining to the distal small intestine

51. Condition where certain sounds elicit a subjective sensation of color

54. Sweats

56. Male ejaculatory fluid

57. One of the components of a whole

58. The outer covering of an organ

59. Inflammation of (suffix)

60. Lacrimal gland secretion

61. ____phia; a wasting away

62. A pouch

Down

1. _______phobia; fear of blushing

2. Death

3. Without a breastbone

4. Tumors (suffix)

5. Treat an anatomic structure with a light beam device

6. Acrocephalosyndactyly (abbrev.)

7. Prefix meaning 'three'

8. _____cide; mite-destroying agent

9. A muscle that moves a bone around it's own axis

10. A condition of sexual excitement

11. Stops

12. ______esis; an eruption or rash

15. _____osis; bone mass within a bone

17. The smallest of a litter

19. ___dontia; absence of teeth

23. Abbreviation for International Classification of Diseases

25. Therefore

26. Prefix referring to lips

27. Antistreptolysin-O test (abbrev.)

30. A ridge formed by the doubling back of a lamina

31. ___ectasis; collapsed lung

33. ____onic; having equal tension

34. An abnormal narrowing of a duct

35. Back part of the skull

36. One of a threesome of neck muscles

37. Substance

40. Pertaining to a poisonous vapor

41. A wall of an organ or cavity

42. Occurring every 8th day

44. Soft innermost layer of a tooth

45. Prefix meaning 'with'

47. _____algia; stomach ache

48. _____phobia; fear of returning home

51. ____ract; to extend forward

52. To perceive by the ear

53. Prefix signifying one quadrillion

55. Abbreviation for islet cell antibody

48

Across

1. A-naphthylthiourea (abbrev.)
5. The body of a nerve cell
9. _____algia; sciatica
14. ____cephalon; most recently evolved brain part
15. ____toe; hallux varus
16. _____cholia; a mental depression
17. A sound of distinct frequency
18. The germinated and dried seed of barley
19. Roman 1053
20. Within the cavity of a joint
23. ____caria; hives
24. ___nism; coitus interruptus
25. ______lagnia; sexual gratification through theft
28. Prefix meaning 'eyelash' or 'eyelid'
30. ___algia; pain in a limb
33. _____ cranial nerve; glossopharyngeal
34. Minute opening of the skin
35. Combustible material burned on the skin as a cautery
36. Between the neuromeres
39. Give nourishment to
40. ____itis; blood vessel inflammation
41. _____osis; bone mass within a bone
42. Hearing organ
43. ____uria; normal urination
44. ______lith; dental calculus
45. Roman 700
46. ____adenoma; benign sweat gland tumor
47. An agent that causes vomiting and purging
54. _____cardia; imperfect development of the heart
55. ____tia; resistance to motion, action, or change
56. To restore to health
57. Examinations
58. Refuse to admit
59. Prefix meaning 'within'
60. Irregularly notched, toothed, or indented
61. ____genous; originating outside the organism
62. Antistreptolysin-O test (abbrev.)

Down

1. Prefix meaning 'against'
2. An inert gaseous element in the atmosphere
3. A bed covering for administering oxygen
4. A tooth prior to emergence
5. ______genic; originating in the body
6. _____algia; female gonad pain
7. Denature
8. ____culus; joint
9. ______facient; producing disease protection
10. A saddle-shaped anatomical structure
11. Clinical Laboratory Improvement Amendments (acronym)
12. Pilus
13. ___encephaly; occipital cranial defect, with brain exposed
21. _____algia; joint pain
22. _____ptosis; prolapse of the vagina
25. Cutting tool
26. Line
27. _____algia; intestinal pain
28. To suddenly expel air from the lungs
29. _____gate; to wash out
30. A stupid person
31. To have life
32. _____genesis; milk production
34. ____atomic; denoting five atoms per molecule
35. Excessive menstruation
37. _____lepsy; excessive sleep disorder
38. Tunica _____; middle artery wall layer
43. Sugar containing eight carbon atoms
44. ______genes; related to the eyebrows
45. Short for shoulder muscles
46. A mold for keeping a skin graft in place
47. ____nal; everlasting
48. ____morph; large, strong body type
49. Suffix meaning 'killer'
50. ____dotal; based on case histories
51. Method of reducing pain by electric current (abbrev.)
52. Instrumental activities of daily living (acronym)
53. End result of coagulation
54. Had food

49

1	2	3	4	■	5	6	7	8	9	■	10	11	12	13
14				■	15					■	16			
17				18						19				
20					■	■	21							■
■	■	■	22		23	24	■	25				■	■	■
26	27	28	■	29			30	■	31			32	33	34
35			■	36				37	■	■	38			
39			40						41	42				
43				■	■	44					■	45		
46				47	48	■	49				■	50		
■	■	■	51			52	■	53			54	■	■	■
■	55	56					57	■	■	58		59	60	61
62								63	64					
65				■	66					■	67			
68				■	69					■	70			

Across

1. Big, clumsy people
5. Restores to health
10. ____naceous; soapy
14. A dose of medicine
15. Prefix meaning 'head'
16. ____otomy; incision into an apical structure
17. Relating to occipital bone and mastoid process
20. _____dynia; nose pain
21. To strike or tap firmly
22. White
25. ____sightedness; myopia
26. Abbreviation for dyspnea on exertion
29. Treat with a light beam device
31. Stable, with opposing forces in balance
35. Abbreviation for estrogen replacement therapy
36. Prefix meaning 'within'
38. ____dynia; sinew pain
39. Dwarfism characterized by gross limb shortening and hydropic head and trunk
43. ____itis; tenosynovitis
44. _____gnosia; sensory inattention
45. Short for arm adductor
46. The odor of the axillae
49. Toward the mouth
50. ___pose; fatty
51. ____insic; of internal origin
53. ____eurosis; sheet-like tendon
55. Dies
58. _____algia; bodily pain
62. Stimulating to secretion
65. A manner of walking
66. Whiteheads
67. ____aphobia; fear of public places
68. ____mania; compulsive shopping
69. _____omosis; blood vessel coalescence
70. ____sis; abnormal hunger

Down

1. Smell
2. Superior, aortic curve
3. Central points
4. _____ bifida; vertebral arch fusion failure
5. Hydrochloric acid (abbrev.)
6. Consume
7. ____tosis; cell suicide
8. A threshold or boundary
9. Looks intently
10. Soak
11. ____taxis; slight hemorrhage
12. Landmark located below PSIS
13. Abbreviation for obsessive-compulsive disorder
18. ______osis; hay fever
19. ____emia; intestinal autointoxication
23. ____age; dressing holder
24. _____phobia; fear of thunderstorms
26. The cessation of life
27. _____algia; pain in the testes
28. Used as an early anaesthetic
30. _____genic; causing sexual arousal
32. SI unit of magnetic flux density
33. In a direction toward the inion
34. _____form; rib-shaped
37. _____phobia; fear of public places
40. Prefix referring to the back of the head
41. Abbreviation for expiratory positive airway pressure
42. Having many projections or protuberances
47. One of the components of a whole
48. Supporting framework of an organ
52. An organic substance, insoluble in water
54. Dorsal
55. ____thropic; originating outside the human body
56. Roman 92
57. ____phobia; fear of light flashes
59. ____lalia; pathological speech problem
60. Active range of motion (abbrev.)
61. ____genous; originating in cheese
62. The self
63. Abbreviation for carcinoma in situ
64. Disease-spreading rodent

50

Across

1. Fetor ____; halitosis
5. ____naceous; soapy
9. _____phobia; fear of eating
14. ____fibrosis; phlebosclerosis
15. Community mental health center (acronym)
16. _____lycemia; abnormally low blood sugar level
17. Within the heart muscle
20. Nostrils
21. Small, raised bone eminence
22. A yellow scleroprotein
25. ___itis; inflammation of gastric cellular tissue
26. _____dynia; breast pain
28. ____taxis; slight hemorrhage
32. Pertaining to deficiency of blood
37. A dry, thin flake of epidermis
38. Relating to the external ear and skull
41. Medicine doses
42. Organ joining mother and fetus
43. ____itude; a sense of weariness
44. A sonorous and convulsive inspiration
46. ___cardia; systole
47. Recurring every 3rd day
53. Toward the head
58. _____schisis; cleft palate
59. Dwarfism characterized by gross limb shortening and hydropic head and trunk
62. _____form; cartwheel-patterned
63. ____osis; a bodily passage narrowing
64. To act out with gestures and body movement
65. Amyo_____; muscle tone defect
66. Abbreviation for eye, ear, nose, and throat
67. Abbreviation for obstructive sleep apnea syndrome

Down

1. Relating to sheep
2. Referring to the kidney
3. Prefix meaning 'within'
4. Open skin lesions
5. Head flexor (abbrev.)
6. ___ous; lacking muscular tissue
7. ____esthesis; light sensitivity
8. Obscured or concealed
9. _____algia; pain in the diaphragm
10. ____emia; excess water in the blood
11. ____otomy; incision into an apex
12. Any objective an organism seeks to attain
13. To eye provocatively
18. Aspartate aminotransferase (abbrev.)
19. ____genesis; development of life from nonlife
23. ____nogen; antigen
24. Protective cover on the dorsal distal phalanges
27. _____philia; voyeurism
28. Breakout of pimples
29. Ache
30. Abbreviation for other licensed antifungal therapies
31. ____phobia; fear of light flashes
32. Abbreviation for instrumental activities of daily living
33. The calf
34. Acronym for contralateral routing of signal
35. Coxae
36. Abbreviation for electrocerebral silence
37. A pouch
39. End result of coagulation
40. Forceful, unconsentual sexual intercourse
44. Living in a natural state
45. Having a noisy voice
46. Dipso_____; alcoholism
48. Move swiftly on foot
49. _____phobia; fear of involuntarily shaking
50. Arsen_____; chronic arsenic poisoning
51. The soul or life
52. Olfactory organs
53. Protective plaster shell
54. ____genous; originating outside the organism
55. A unit of apparent loudness
56. ____zontal; perpendicular to the vertical
57. Anti____; poison-stopping substance
60. ___eric; nonproprietary
61. Abbreviation for ears, nose, and throat

Medi-Cross II

ANSWERS

1

L	A	X	A		P	I	L	A	R		G	A	M	O
I	N	E	R		U	R	I	N	E		A	N	A	B
F	E	R	R		P	I	V	O	T		L	I	N	E
E	C	O	E	P	I	D	E	M	I	O	L	O	G	Y
			C	H	L	O	R			B	O	N	E	S
O	T	I	T	I	S			L	I	E	N			
P	O	N	O			S	H	I	N	S		M	R	A
I	N	T	R	A	E	P	I	T	H	E	L	I	A	L
A	E	R		F	L	U	S	H			A	L	G	A
			U	T	E	R			P	A	C	K	E	R
T	A	S	T	E			S	C	O	L	E			
I	N	T	E	R	M	E	T	A	C	A	R	P	A	L
D	I	A	R		A	L	E	U	K		T	O	P	O
A	M	B	U		S	E	N	S	E		U	R	I	C
L	A	S	S		O	C	T	E	T		S	I	C	K

2

H	U	M	S			C	O	G		O	C	T	A	D
E	T	E	C		S	O	R	E		G	L	E	N	O
M	E	A	L		P	L	A	N		L	I	N	E	R
A	R	T	E	R	I	O	L	O	V	E	N	O	U	S
			R	A	T	S			I	S	I			
A	N	I	O	N	S		I	E	P		C	E	L	O
S	O	L	I	D		O	S	T	E	M		M	I	D
I	R	I	D	O	S	C	L	E	R	O	T	O	M	Y
A	M	A		M	A	T	E	R		R	E	T	I	N
L	O	C	I		C	O	T		A	T	R	E	T	O
			A	B	R			A	N	A	M			
G	A	S	T	R	O	E	N	T	E	R	I	T	I	S
A	G	O	R	A		H	A	R	M		N	O	C	T
I	O	N	I	C		E	T	I	O		A	C	H	E
T	R	O	C	H		C	R	O			L	O	O	P

3

R	A	M	I		F	E	T	A	L		P	A	R	O
O	N	Y	M		A	R	E	N	A		A	N	A	B
L	E	S	B		M	O	R	O	N		L	I	N	E
E	C	O	E	P	I	D	E	M	I	O	L	O	G	Y
			C	A	N	E	S			B	O	N	E	S
P	H	R	I	N	E			A	B	E	R			
H	E	A	L			P	I	L	L	S		A	D	P
A	R	T	E	R	I	O	L	O	V	E	N	O	U	S
C	O	S		U	L	N	A	E			I	R	R	I
			A	B	I	O			R	E	C	T	A	L
P	H	O	N	O			G	N	O	T	O			
H	Y	P	E	R	P	A	R	A	S	I	T	I	S	M
A	P	E	R		A	L	A	R	A		I	D	E	O
C	O	N	G		L	A	S	E	R		N	E	A	R
O	P	S	Y		L	E	P	S	Y		E	A	T	S

4

L	A	C	E	R		E	M	G		O	V	U	L	A
A	L	A	R	A		F	U	O		V	I	N	I	C
C	O	L	O	P		F	R	I	C	A	T	I	V	E
T	E	C	T	I		E	M	T	A	L	A			
		A	I	D		C	U	R	L		M	E	A	T
C	I	R	C		A	T	R	O			I	N	T	E
A	N	I		A	P	O	S		T	E	N	D	O	N
S	H	U	D	D	E	R		P	E	R	S	O	N	S
E	A	R	W	A	X		P	E	L	V		M	I	O
I	L	I	A			P	E	R	O		T	E	A	R
N	E	A	R		C	H	E	M		A	R	T		
			F	E	M	A	L	E		N	A	R	C	O
H	E	M	I	A	L	G	I	A		A	N	I	O	N
E	X	I	S	T		I	N	T		S	C	A	L	A
P	A	L	M	S		A	G	E		T	E	L	E	N

5

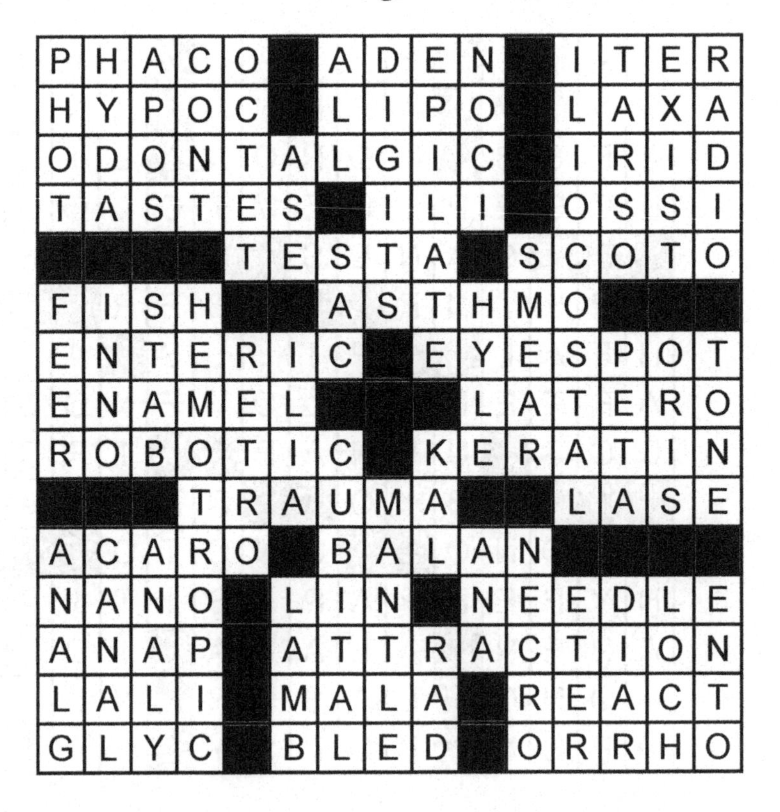

6

L	A	C	T	O		C	A	N	E		H	A	N	D
A	D	R	E	N		A	N	E	U		E	N	U	R
N	E	U	R	A		S	C	A	R		M	E	T	O
I	N	S	A	N	I	T	A	R	Y		I	C	R	P
				I	N	R			O	R	C	H	I	S
	F	L	A	S	H		H	E	P	A	R			
I	L	I	U	M		H	E	S	I	T	A	T	E	S
P	E	N	T		C	O	L	I	C		N	O	X	A
V	A	G	O	L	Y	S	I	S		P	I	X	E	L
			L	A	T	E	X		B	R	A	I	N	
S	P	L	E	N	O			O	T	O				
T	E	A	S		C	O	R	R	U	G	A	T	O	R
U	N	C	I		I	T	E	R		E	N	E	M	A
M	I	T	O		D	I	S	H		N	A	N	N	Y
P	A	I	N		E	C	T	O		Y	P	S	I	L

7

A	P	A	P		S	C	A	T			T	A	L	I
N	A	N	O		P	O	R	E	S		E	I	E	C
T	I	T	S		A	L	G	A	E		M	I	N	D
A	N	E	T	O		D	Y	S	P	E	P	S	I	A
		C	U	N	E		R	E	T	R	O			
O	P	E	R	A	N	T		S	A	C	R	A	L	
P	U	D	E	N	D	A	L			P	O	L	Y	O
H	B	E			S	P	A	C	E			I	S	M
R	E	N	A	L			C	A	L	C	E	M	I	A
	S	T	R	E	S	S		D	E	P	R	E	S	S
			I	C	T	E	R		C	A	R	N		
E	M	O	T	I	O	N	A	L		P	A	T	H	O
P	I	T	H		M	I	N	O	R		T	A	I	L
A	T	O	M		A	L	G	I	A		I	R	R	E
P	E	R	O			E	E	N	T		C	Y	T	O

8

M	E	D	I		L	I	V	E	R		A	N	A	B
E	X	O	N		U	R	I	N	E		C	E	R	U
N	A	R	C		C	O	P	E	S		N	O	S	T
I	N	S	U	L	I	N	E	M	I	A		N	E	T
S	T	A	R	E			R	A	S	H		A	N	O
C	H	L		V	A	G			T	A	C	T	I	C
			A	I	C	H	M	O			P	A	C	K
		E	N	T	E	R	O	R	E	N	A	L		
T	E	X	T			H	I	C	C	U	P			
A	N	H	I	D	R			H	O	M		C	T	A
C	L	A		D	O	T	E			B	A	L	A	N
T	A	L		S	T	E	T	H	O	S	C	O	P	E
U	R	I	C		A	T	H	E	R		A	N	O	M
A	G	N	O		T	R	E	A	T		R	E	T	I
L	E	G	S		E	A	R	T	H		I	D	E	A

9

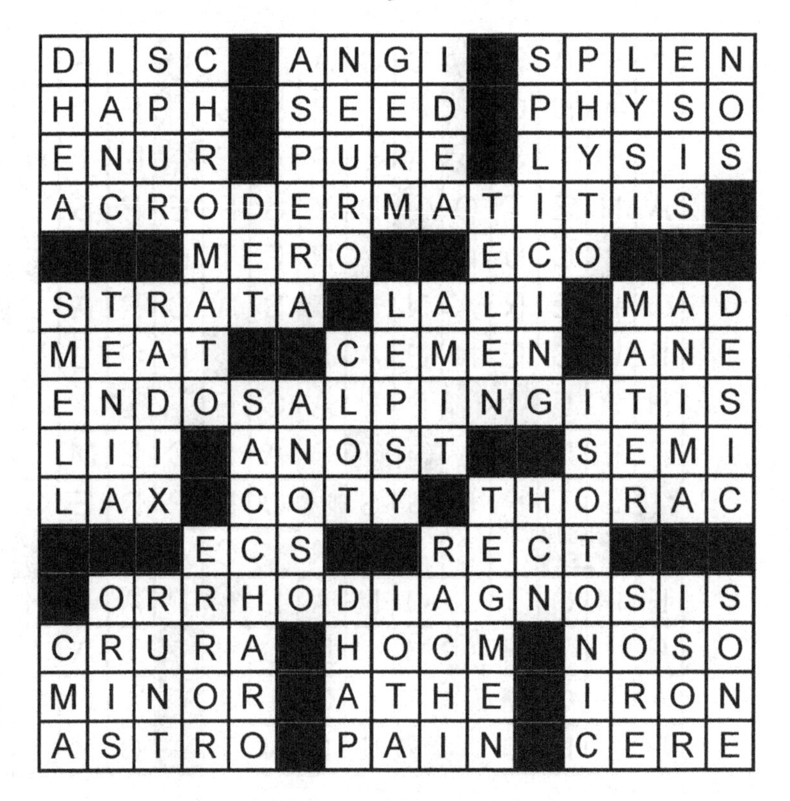

D	I	S	C		A	N	G	I		S	P	L	E	N
H	A	P	H		S	E	E	D		P	H	Y	S	O
E	N	U	R		P	U	R	E		L	Y	S	I	S
A	C	R	O	D	E	R	M	A	T	I	T	I	S	
			M	E	R	O			E	C	O			
S	T	R	A	T	A		L	A	L	I		M	A	D
M	E	A	T			C	E	M	E	N		A	N	E
E	N	D	O	S	A	L	P	I	N	G	I	T	I	S
L	I	I		A	N	O	S	T			S	E	M	I
L	A	X		C	O	T	Y		T	H	O	R	A	C
			E	C	S			R	E	C	T			
	O	R	R	H	O	D	I	A	G	N	O	S	I	S
C	R	U	R	A		H	O	C	M		N	O	S	O
M	I	N	O	R		A	T	H	E		I	R	O	N
A	S	T	R	O		P	A	I	N		C	E	R	E

10

A	C	H	E	S		V	A	G	I		L	A	C	E
C	H	O	L	O		E	P	A	P		A	N	O	X
H	E	M	A	N	G	I	O	S	A	R	C	O	M	A
E	M	O	T	I	O	N	S			H	U	M	A	N
			I	C	A			S	H	I	N			
H	A	L	O		L	A	C	T	I	N	A	T	E	D
A	L	A	N			T	O	R	S	O		A	C	E
A	G	C			H	Y	D	A	T			B	H	N
R	O	T		D	E	P	O	T			S	L	I	T
T	R	I	G	E	M	I	N	A	L		T	E	N	O
			A	R	E	A			I	S	I			
H	I	L	U	M			N	O	S	T	R	I	L	S
O	L	I	G	O	Z	O	O	S	P	E	R	M	I	A
M	I	T	E		E	N	D	S		P	U	P	I	L
I	A	H	S		A	C	E	I		S	P	L	I	T

11

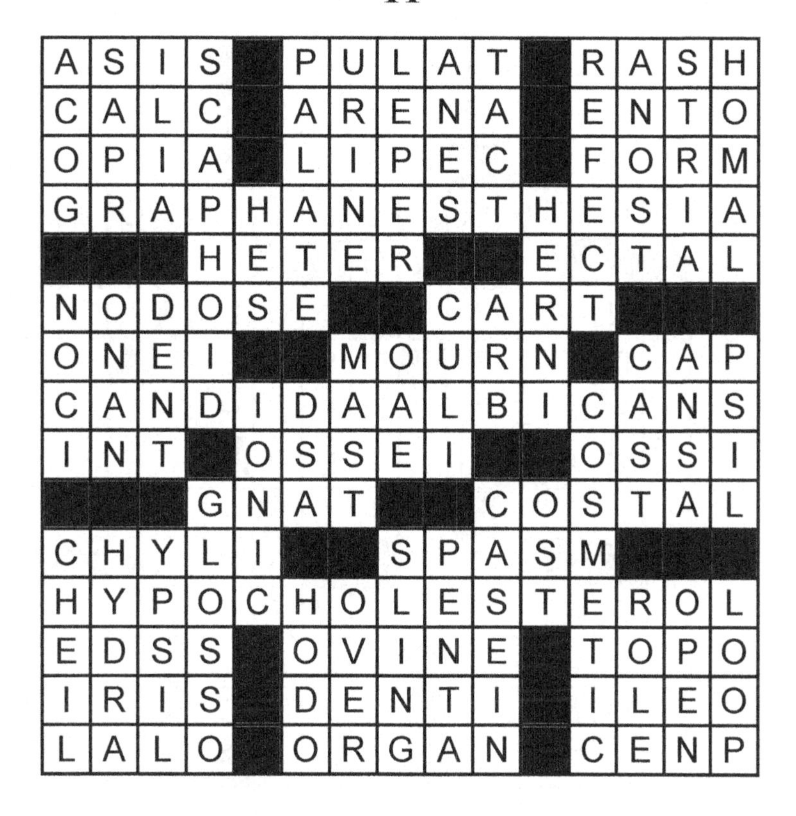

A	S	I	S		P	U	L	A	T		R	A	S	H
C	A	L	C		A	R	E	N	A		E	N	T	O
O	P	I	A		L	I	P	E	C		F	O	R	M
G	R	A	P	H	A	N	E	S	T	H	E	S	I	A
			H	E	T	E	R			E	C	T	A	L
N	O	D	O	S	E			C	A	R	T			
O	N	E	I			M	O	U	R	N		C	A	P
C	A	N	D	I	D	A	A	L	B	I	C	A	N	S
I	N	T		O	S	S	E	I			O	S	S	I
			G	N	A	T			C	O	S	T	A	L
C	H	Y	L	I			S	P	A	S	M			
H	Y	P	O	C	H	O	L	E	S	T	E	R	O	L
E	D	S	S		O	V	I	N	E		T	O	P	O
I	R	I	S		D	E	N	T	I		I	L	E	O
L	A	L	O		O	R	G	A	N		C	E	N	P

12

I	C	A			H	E	A	T	S		V	I	A	L
T	O	N	E		O	N	S	E	T		O	N	C	O
C	P	A	P		M	O	L	A	R		L	I	N	G
H	E	M	I	G	A	S	T	R	E	C	T	O	M	Y
			M	E	L	T			S	Y	S			
S	P	H	E	N	O		K	I	S	S		E	U	R
C	H	I	N			P	I	V	O	T		P	R	E
H	Y	P	O	C	H	O	N	D	R	I	A	S	I	S
I	T	P		L	I	N	E	A			C	O	N	T
Z	O	O		E	D	S	S		V	E	R	M	I	S
			G	F	R			B	E	T	A			
H	E	P	A	T	O	C	A	R	C	I	N	O	M	A
A	X	I	L		S	O	M	A	T		I	R	O	N
R	O	L	E		I	R	I	D	O		A	C	V	D
P	N	E	A		S	A	T	Y	R			H	E	R

13

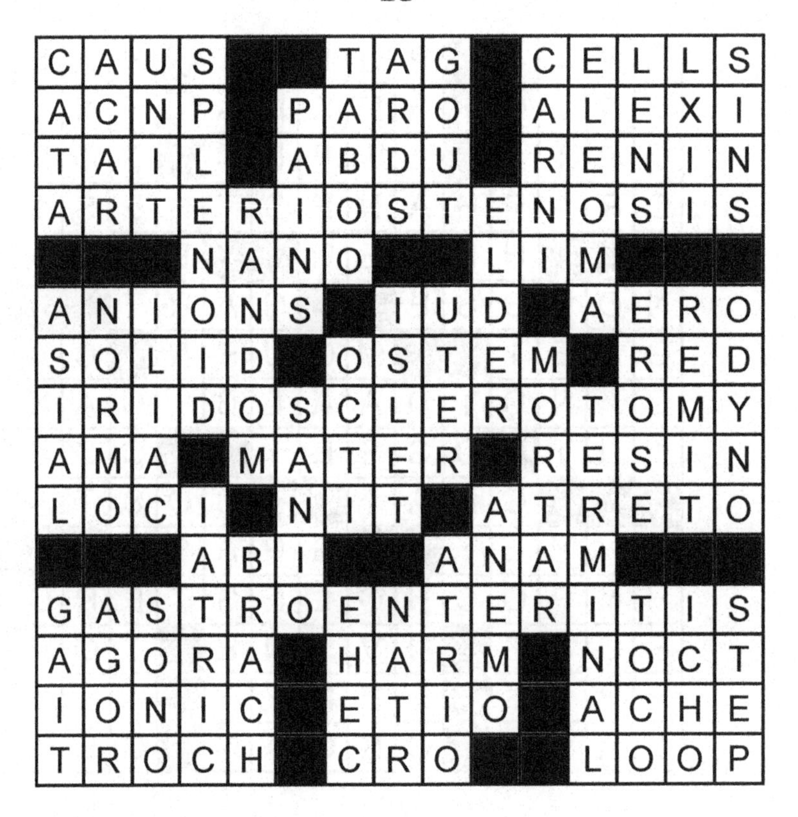
CAUS TAG CELLS
ACNP PARO ALEXI
TAIL ABDU RENIN
ARTERIOSTENOSIS
NANO LIM
ANIONS IUD AERO
SOLID OSTEM RED
IRIDOSCLEROTOMY
AMA MATER RESIN
LOCI NIT ATRETO
ABI ANAM
GASTROENTERITIS
AGORA HARM NOCT
IONIC ETIO ACHE
TROCH CRO LOOP

14

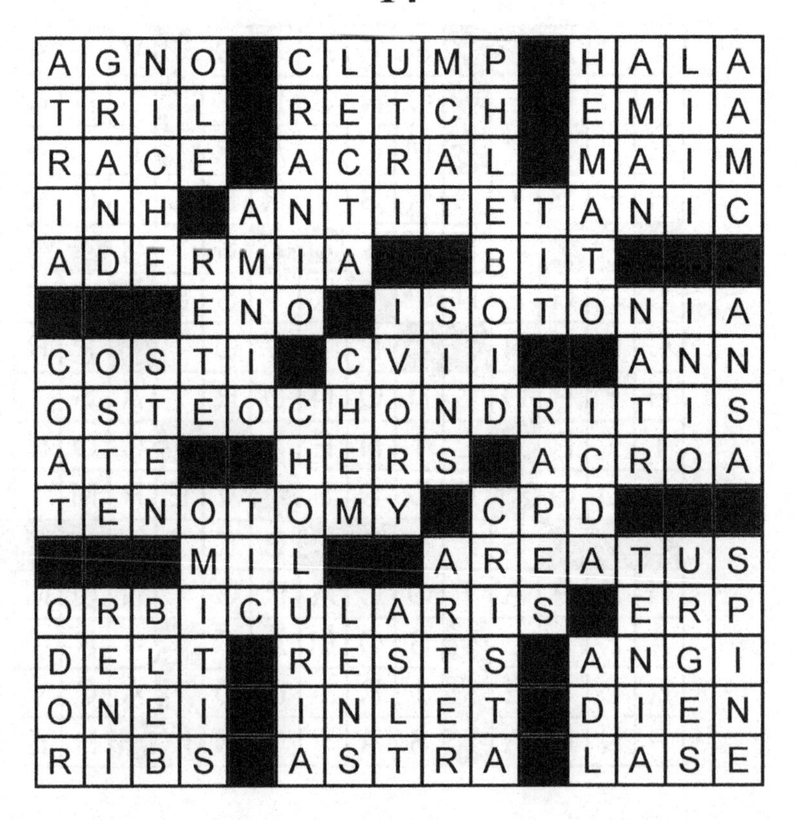
AGNO CLUMP HALA
TRIL RETCH EMIA
RACE ACRAL MAIM
INH ANTITETANIC
ADERMIA BIT
ENO ISOTONIA
COSTI CVII ANN
OSTEOCHONDRITIS
ATE HERS ACROA
TENOTOMY CPD
MIL AREATUS
ORBICULARIS ERP
DELT RESTS ANGI
ONEI INLET DIEN
RIBS ASTRA LASE

15

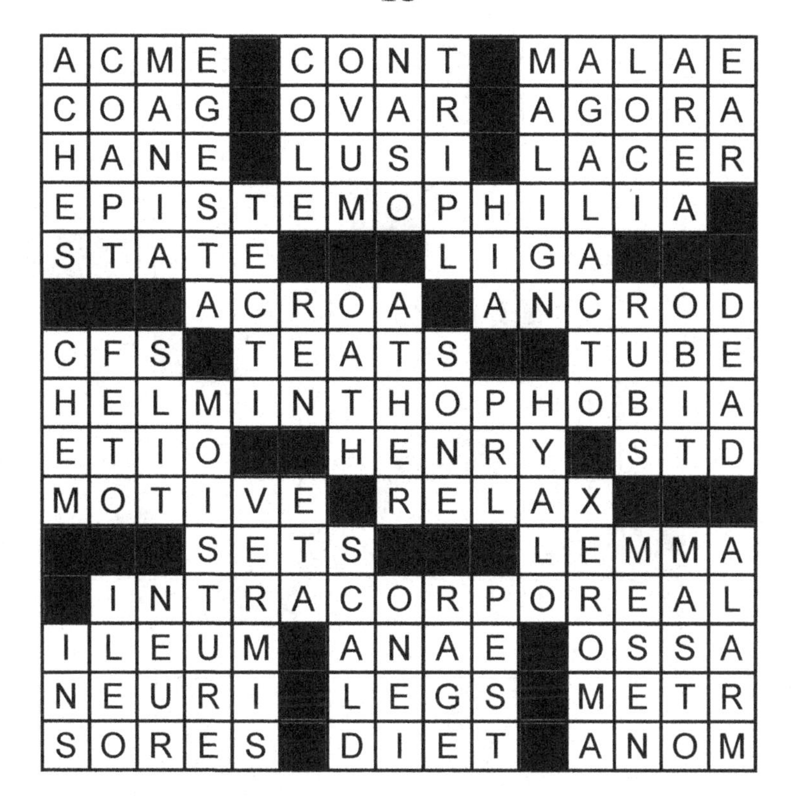
ACME CONT MALAE
COAG OVAR AGORA
HANE LUSI LACER
EPISTEMOPHILIA
STATE LIGA
ACROA ANCROD
CFS TEATS TUBE
HELMINTHOPHOBIA
ETIO HENRY STD
MOTIVE RELAX
SETS LEMMA
INTRACORPOREAL
ILEUM ANAE OSSA
NEURI LEGS METR
SORES DIET ANOM

16

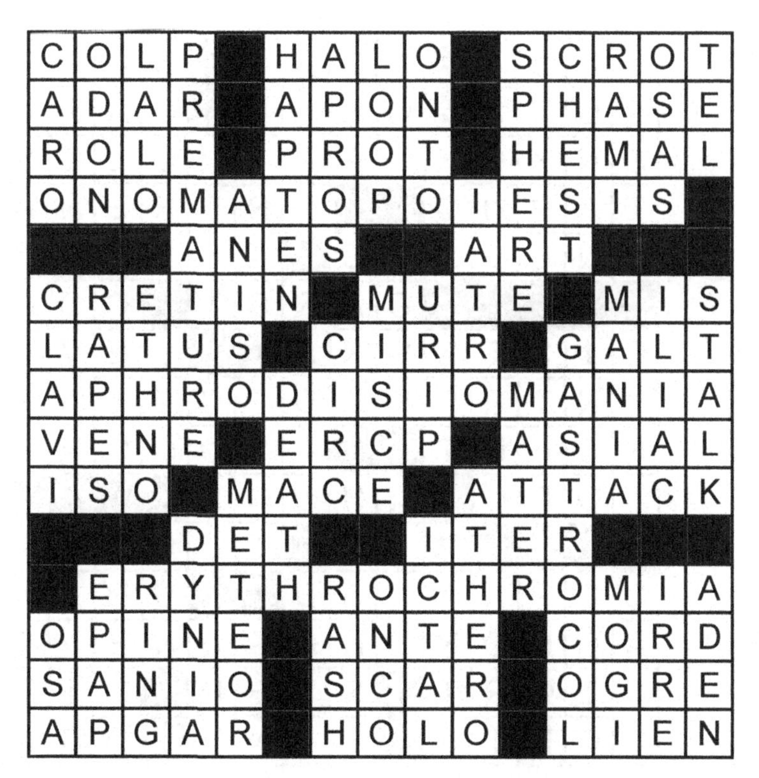
COLP HALO SCROT
ADAR APON PHASE
ROLE PROT HEMAL
ONOMATOPOIESIS
ANES ART
CRETIN MUTE MIS
LATUS CIRR GALT
APHRODISIOMANIA
VENE ERCP ASIAL
ISO MACE ATTACK
DET ITER
ERYTHROCHROMIA
OPINE ANTE CORD
SANIO SCAR OGRE
APGAR HOLO LIEN

17

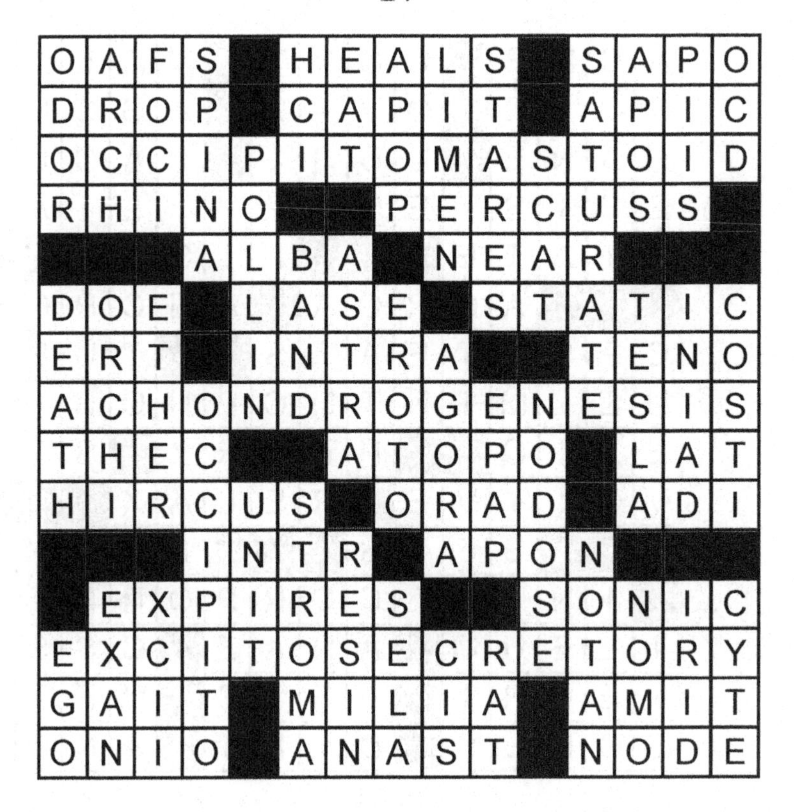

O	A	F	S	#	H	E	A	L	S	#	S	A	P	O
D	R	O	P	#	C	A	P	I	T	#	A	P	I	C
O	C	C	I	P	I	T	O	M	A	S	T	O	I	D
R	H	I	N	O	#	#	P	E	R	C	U	S	S	#
#	#	#	A	L	B	A	#	N	E	A	R	#	#	#
D	O	E	#	L	A	S	E	#	S	T	A	T	I	C
E	R	T	#	I	N	T	R	A	#	#	T	E	N	O
A	C	H	O	N	D	R	O	G	E	N	E	S	I	S
T	H	E	C	#	#	A	T	O	P	O	#	L	A	T
H	I	R	C	U	S	#	O	R	A	D	#	A	D	I
#	#	#	I	N	T	R	#	A	P	O	N	#	#	#
#	E	X	P	I	R	E	S	#	#	S	O	N	I	C
E	X	C	I	T	O	S	E	C	R	E	T	O	R	Y
G	A	I	T	#	M	I	L	I	A	#	A	M	I	T
O	N	I	O	#	A	N	A	S	T	#	N	O	D	E

18

E	N	S	I	#	A	C	A	R	#	S	C	A	R	S
R	O	T	S	#	G	E	N	E	#	C	A	P	U	T
O	N	Y	C	H	O	P	A	T	H	O	L	O	G	Y
T	A	P	H	O	#	#	P	R	E	R	E	N	A	L
O	N	E	I	R	I	C	#	A	S	E	#	#	#	#
#	#	#	#	#	C	A	R	D	I	#	C	O	R	A
C	I	S	T	E	R	N	A	#	#	L	E	V	E	R
I	N	T	E	R	P	E	D	I	C	U	L	A	T	E
S	C	E	N	T	#	#	I	S	O	C	O	R	I	A
T	O	P	O	#	W	H	O	O	P	#	#	#	#	#
#	#	#	#	M	I	O	#	T	E	R	T	I	A	N
C	E	P	H	A	L	A	D	#	#	U	R	A	N	O
A	C	H	O	N	D	R	O	G	E	N	E	S	I	S
S	T	O	R	I	#	S	T	E	N	#	M	I	M	E
T	O	N	I	A	#	E	E	N	T	#	O	S	A	S

19

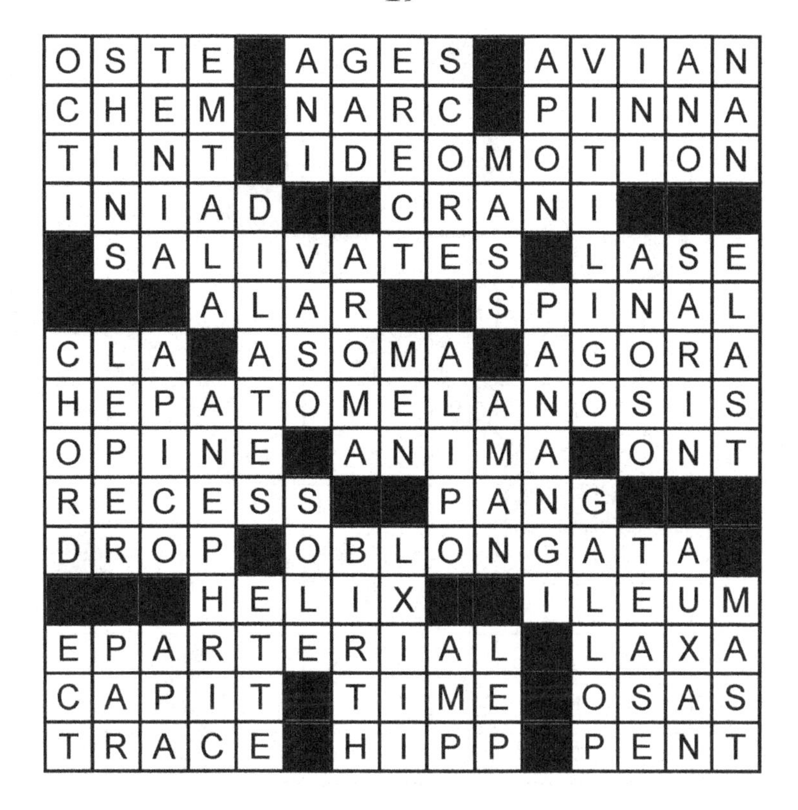

O	S	T	E		A	G	E	S		A	V	I	A	N
C	H	E	M		N	A	R	C		P	I	N	N	A
T	I	N	T		I	D	E	O	M	O	T	I	O	N
I	N	I	A	D			C	R	A	N	I			
	S	A	L	I	V	A	T	E	S		L	A	S	E
			A	L	A	R			S	P	I	N	A	L
C	L	A		A	S	O	M	A		A	G	O	R	A
H	E	P	A	T	O	M	E	L	A	N	O	S	I	S
O	P	I	N	E		A	N	I	M	A		O	N	T
R	E	C	E	S	S			P	A	N	G			
D	R	O	P		O	B	L	O	N	G	A	T	A	
			H	E	L	I	X			I	L	E	U	M
E	P	A	R	T	E	R	I	A	L		L	A	X	A
C	A	P	I	T		T	I	M	E		O	S	A	S
T	R	A	C	E		H	I	P	P		P	E	N	T

20

C	L	I	A		L	A	C	T	I			I	T	P
H	I	N	D		A	G	O	R	A		I	D	E	O
I	N	T	R	A	P	E	R	I	T	O	N	E	A	L
L	E	I		C	A	N	A	L		P	L	A	T	E
L	A	M	B	E	R	T			H	E	E	L	S	
		I	L	I	O		S	H	O	R	T			
G	A	T	E			A	C	A	R	O		P	H	I
A	R	I	B	O	F	L	A	V	I	N	O	S	I	S
P	E	S		S	I	G	N	S			P	O	R	I
			A	T	L	A	S		A	P	E	R		
	M	E	T	R	A			C	R	A	N	I	A	L
N	I	C	H	E		S	T	O	R	I		A	M	A
O	S	T	E	O	A	N	A	G	E	N	E	S	I	S
S	C	A	R		P	A	I	N	S		P	I	N	E
T	E	L			S	P	L	I	T		I	S	O	R

21

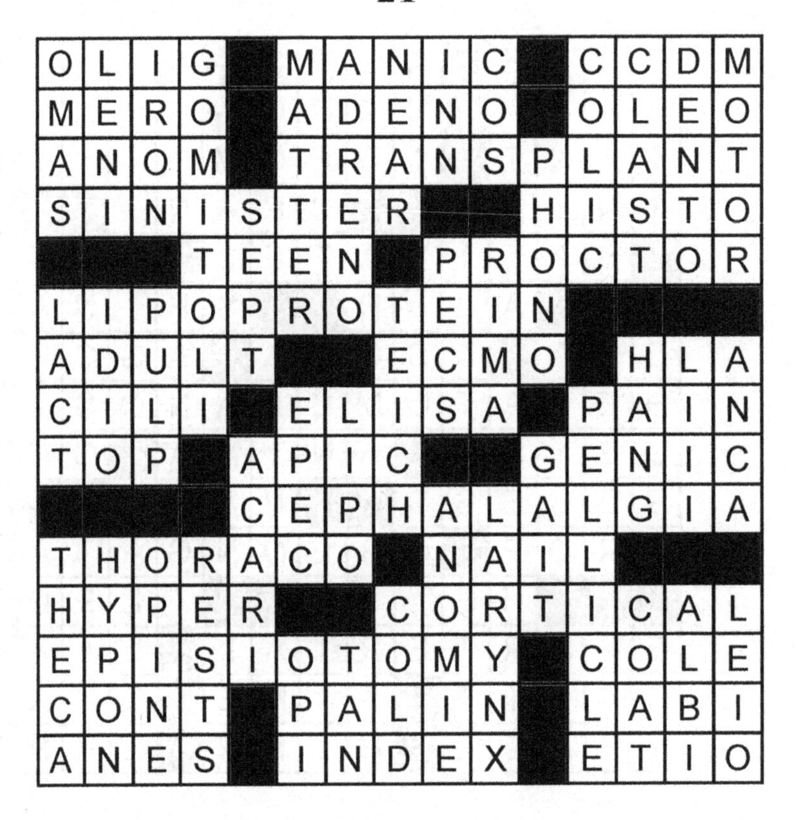
OLIG MANIC CCDM
MERO ADENO OLEO
ANOM TRANSPLANT
SINISTER HISTO
TEEN PROCTOR
LIPOPROTEIN
ADULT ECMO HLA
CILI ELISA PAIN
TOP APIC GENIC
CEPHALALGIA
THORACO NAIL
HYPER CORTICAL
EPISIOTOMY COLE
CONT PALIN LABI
ANES INDEX ETIO

22

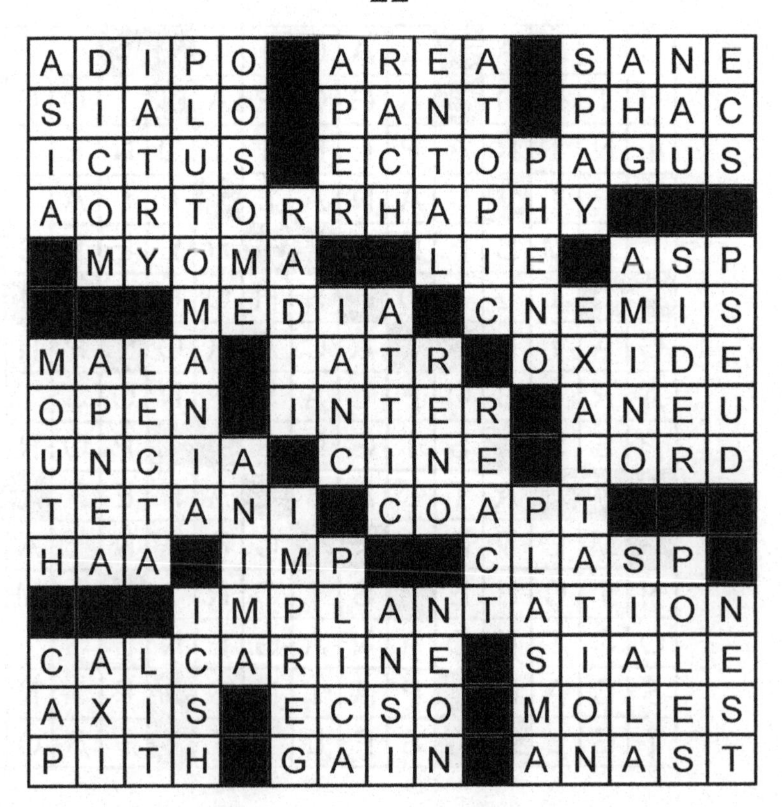
ADIPO AREA SANE
SIALO PANT PHAC
ICTUS ECTOPAGUS
AORTORRHAPHY
MYOMA LIE ASP
MEDIA CNEMIS
MALA IATR OXIDE
OPEN INTER ANEU
UNCIA CINE LORD
TETANI COAPT
HAA IMP CLASP
IMPLANTATION
CALCARINE SIALE
AXIS ECSO MOLES
PITH GAIN ANAST

23

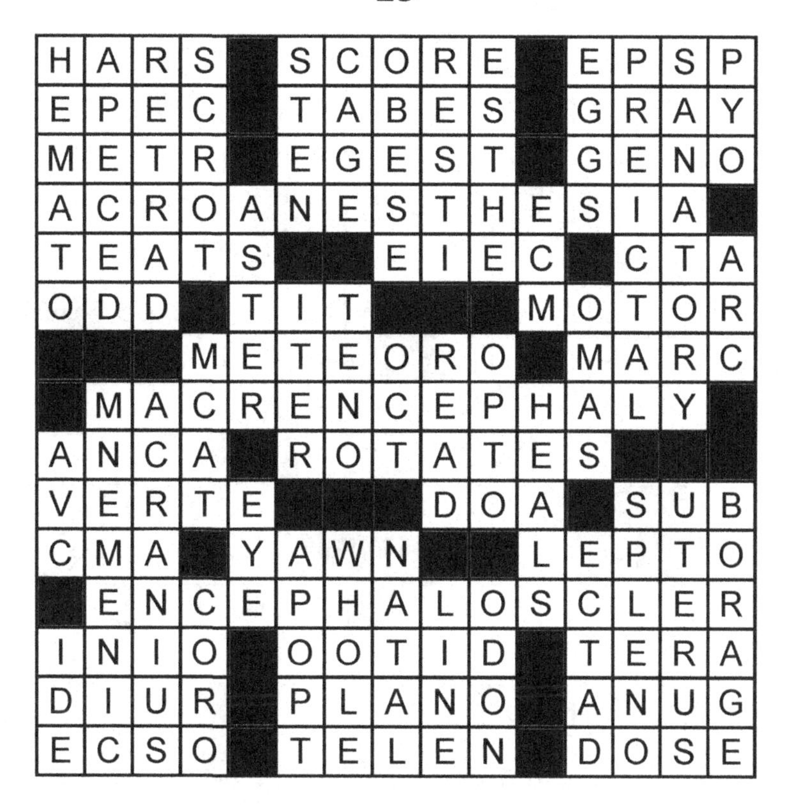

H	A	R	S		S	C	O	R	E		E	P	S	P
E	P	E	C		T	A	B	E	S		G	R	A	Y
M	E	T	R		E	G	E	S	T		G	E	N	O
A	C	R	O	A	N	E	S	T	H	E	S	I	A	
T	E	A	T	S			E	I	E	C		C	T	A
O	D	D		T	I	T				M	O	T	O	R
			M	E	T	E	O	R	O		M	A	R	C
	M	A	C	R	E	N	C	E	P	H	A	L	Y	
A	N	C	A		R	O	T	A	T	E	S			
V	E	R	T	E				D	O	A		S	U	B
C	M	A		Y	A	W	N			L	E	P	T	O
	E	N	C	E	P	H	A	L	O	S	C	L	E	R
I	N	I	O		O	O	T	I	D		T	E	R	A
D	I	U	R		P	L	A	N	O		A	N	U	G
E	C	S	O		T	E	L	E	N		D	O	S	E

24

C	A	V	A		W	A	V	E		A	S	T	R	A
A	M	A	N		A	G	E	S		S	T	A	I	N
L	A	S	E		S	O	N	O		P	A	L	M	S
C	L	A	U	S	T	R	O	P	H	O	B	I	A	
				C	E	A		H	E	R	S			
E	N	E	M	A	S		T	O	P	O		A	A	V
L	O	C	A	L		C	O	R	A		A	N	C	A
I	N	T	R	A	P	E	R	I	T	O	N	E	A	L
S	A	R	C		A	N	T	A		N	A	T	R	I
A	N	O		A	R	T	I		C	Y	T	O	I	D
			S	P	U	R		C	O	C				
	A	R	T	E	R	I	O	R	R	H	A	P	H	Y
F	L	O	O	R		O	R	A	D		A	N	A	E
A	B	O	R	T		L	I	N	I		S	E	L	A
R	A	T	I	O		E	S	I	S		H	A	I	R

25

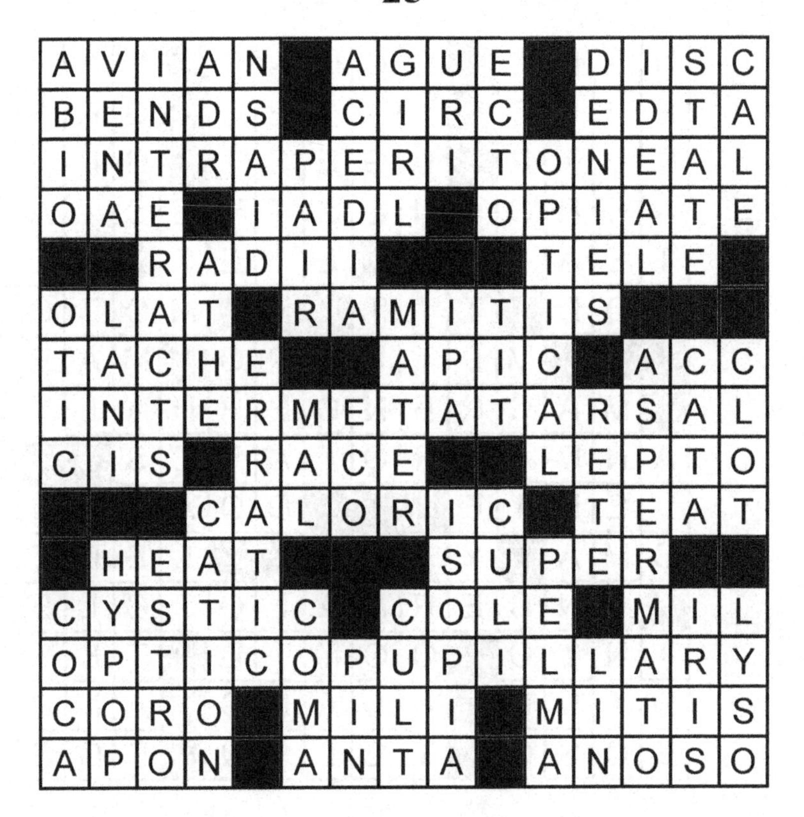

A	V	I	A	N		A	G	U	E		D	I	S	C
B	E	N	D	S		C	I	R	C		E	D	T	A
I	N	T	R	A	P	E	R	I	T	O	N	E	A	L
O	A	E		I	A	D	L		O	P	I	A	T	E
		R	A	D	I	I				T	E	L	E	
O	L	A	T		R	A	M	I	T	I	S			
T	A	C	H	E			A	P	I	C		A	C	C
I	N	T	E	R	M	E	T	A	T	A	R	S	A	L
C	I	S		R	A	C	E			L	E	P	T	O
			C	A	L	O	R	I	C		T	E	A	T
	H	E	A	T				S	U	P	E	R		
C	Y	S	T	I	C		C	O	L	E		M	I	L
O	P	T	I	C	O	P	U	P	I	L	L	A	R	Y
C	O	R	O		M	I	L	I		M	I	T	I	S
A	P	O	N		A	N	T	A		A	N	O	S	O

26

I	P	S	P		S	P	A	C	E		O	C	T	I
D	I	P	L		T	Y	P	E	S		C	O	R	A
A	L	A	E		A	G	E	N	T		C	L	I	T
	I	N	T	E	R	A	R	T	I	C	U	L	A	R
			H	E	E	L			M	A	L	A	D	Y
M	O	R	O	N	S		H	A	A	R	T			
E	V	E	R	T		D	E	N	T	O		A	M	N
L	U	N	A		U	R	A	T	E		O	L	E	O
O	M	O		S	T	O	R	I		P	S	O	A	S
			S	T	E	P	S		P	A	T	E	N	T
D	I	A	P	E	R			P	O	L	E			
O	C	C	I	P	I	T	O	A	T	L	O	I	D	
R	H	I	N		T	E	S	L	A		A	N	E	C
S	O	N	E		I	N	T	I	M		N	O	C	I
O	R	I	S		S	T	E	N	O		A	S	I	S

27

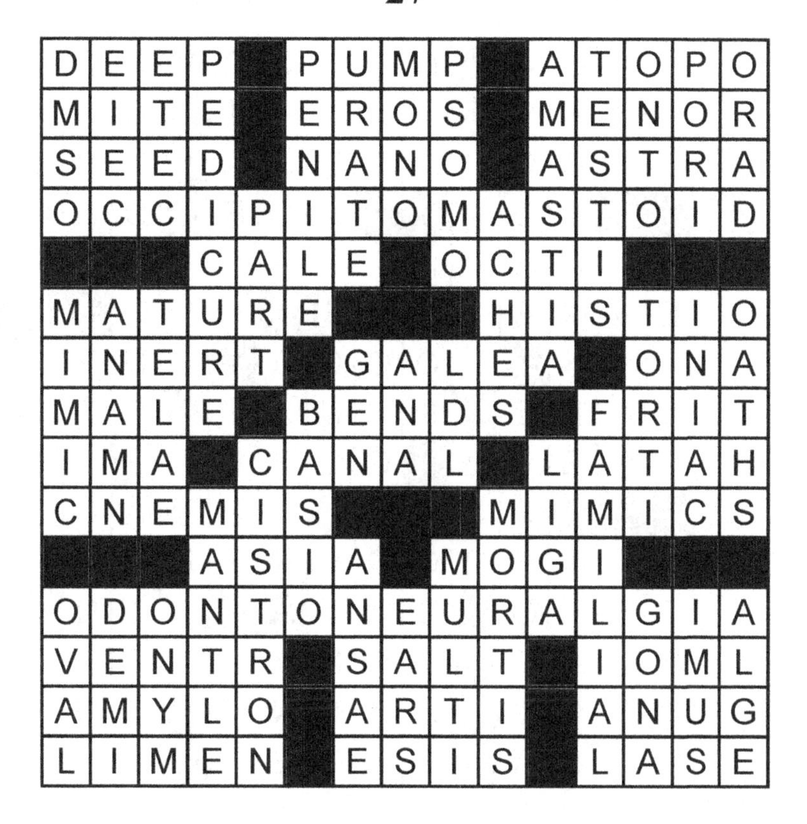

D	E	E	P	#	P	U	M	P	#	A	T	O	P	O
M	I	T	E	#	E	R	O	S	#	M	E	N	O	R
S	E	E	D	#	N	A	N	O	#	A	S	T	R	A
O	C	C	I	P	I	T	O	M	A	S	T	O	I	D
#	#	#	C	A	L	E	#	O	C	T	I	#	#	#
M	A	T	U	R	E	#	#	#	H	I	S	T	I	O
I	N	E	R	T	#	G	A	L	E	A	#	O	N	A
M	A	L	E	#	B	E	N	D	S	#	F	R	I	T
I	M	A	#	C	A	N	A	L	#	L	A	T	A	H
C	N	E	M	I	S	#	#	#	M	I	M	I	C	S
#	#	#	A	S	I	A	#	M	O	G	I	#	#	#
O	D	O	N	T	O	N	E	U	R	A	L	G	I	A
V	E	N	T	R	#	S	A	L	T	#	I	O	M	L
A	M	Y	L	O	#	A	R	T	I	#	A	N	U	G
L	I	M	E	N	#	E	S	I	S	#	L	A	S	E

28

H	E	P	A	#	P	E	N	T	#	#	A	M	A	N
A	T	O	M	#	A	C	A	R	O	#	M	O	N	O
M	E	S	O	T	R	O	P	I	C	#	P	R	O	S
A	R	T	E	R	I	#	E	A	T	#	H	O	S	T
#	#	#	B	A	E	P	#	G	E	R	O	N	T	O
O	L	F	A	C	T	O	M	E	T	E	R	#	#	#
M	I	O	#	T	E	N	O	#	#	M	I	M	I	C
A	N	A	P	#	S	O	N	I	C	#	C	E	L	O
S	E	M	E	N	#	#	A	R	O	M	#	D	I	G
#	#	#	C	O	O	R	D	I	N	A	T	I	O	N
L	A	C	T	O	S	E	#	S	A	N	E	#	#	#
A	T	R	O	#	T	A	P	#	T	I	C	K	L	E
T	E	A	R	#	E	M	A	C	I	A	T	I	O	N
U	L	N	A	#	M	E	T	R	O	#	U	N	I	T
S	O	I	L	#	#	R	H	I	N	#	M	E	N	O

29

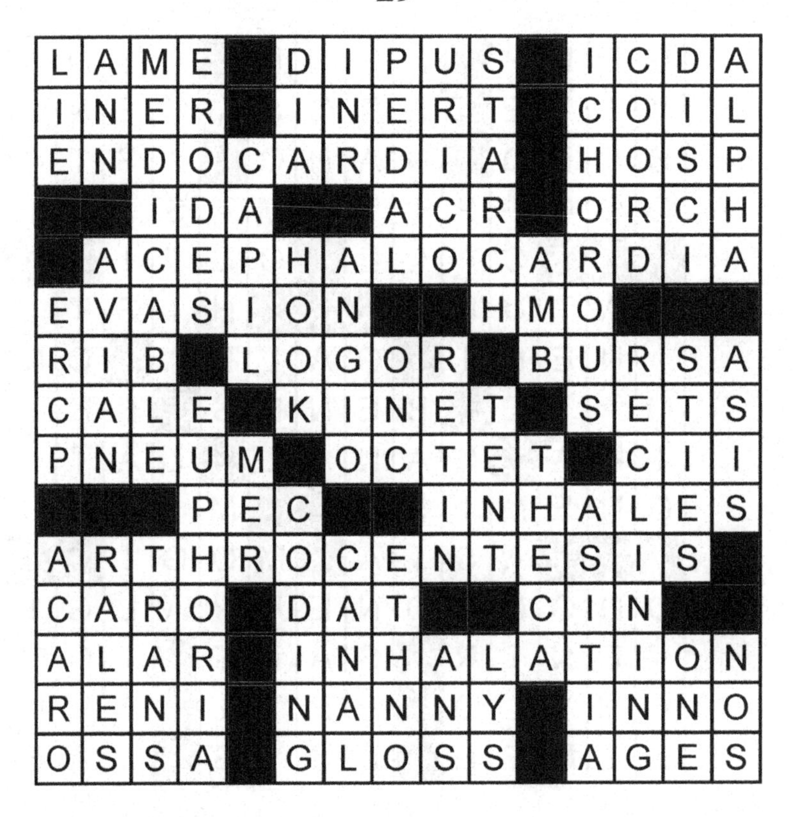

LAME DIPUS ICDA
INER INERT COIL
ENDOCARDIA HOSP
IDA ACR ORCH
ACEPHALOCARDIA
EVASION HMO
RIB LOGOR BURSA
CALE KINET SETS
PNEUM OCTET CII
PEC INHALES
ARTHROCENTESIS
CARO DAT CIN
ALAR INHALATION
RENI NANNY INNO
OSSA GLOSS AGES

30

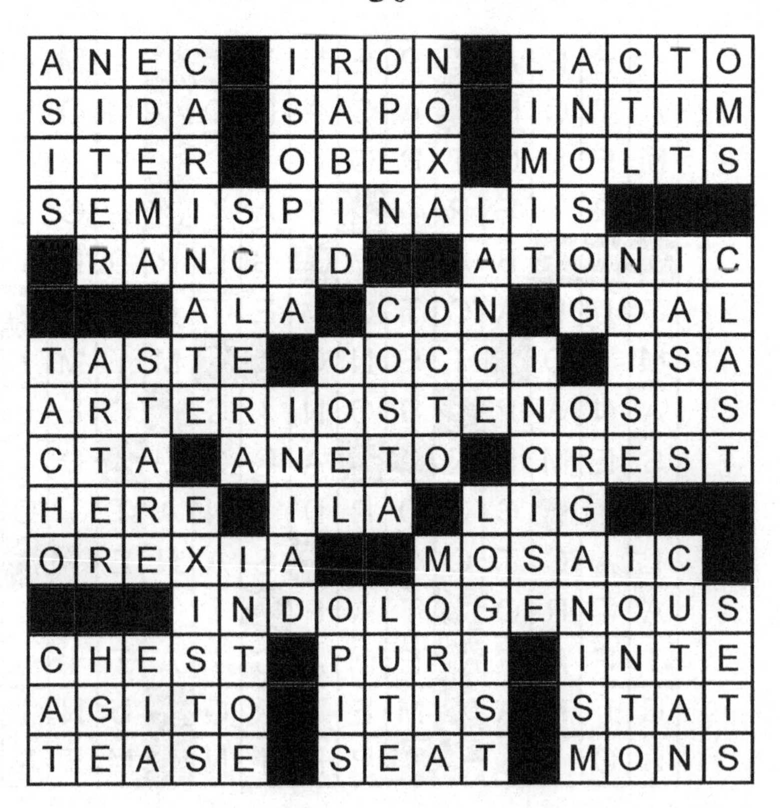

ANEC IRON LACTO
SIDA SAPO INTIM
ITER OBEX MOLTS
SEMISPINALIS
RANCID ATONIC
ALA CON GOAL
TASTE COCCI ISA
ARTERIOSTENOSIS
CTA ANETO CREST
HERE ILA LIG
OREXIA MOSAIC
INDOLOGENOUS
CHEST PURI INTE
AGITO ITIS STAT
TEASE SEAT MONS

31

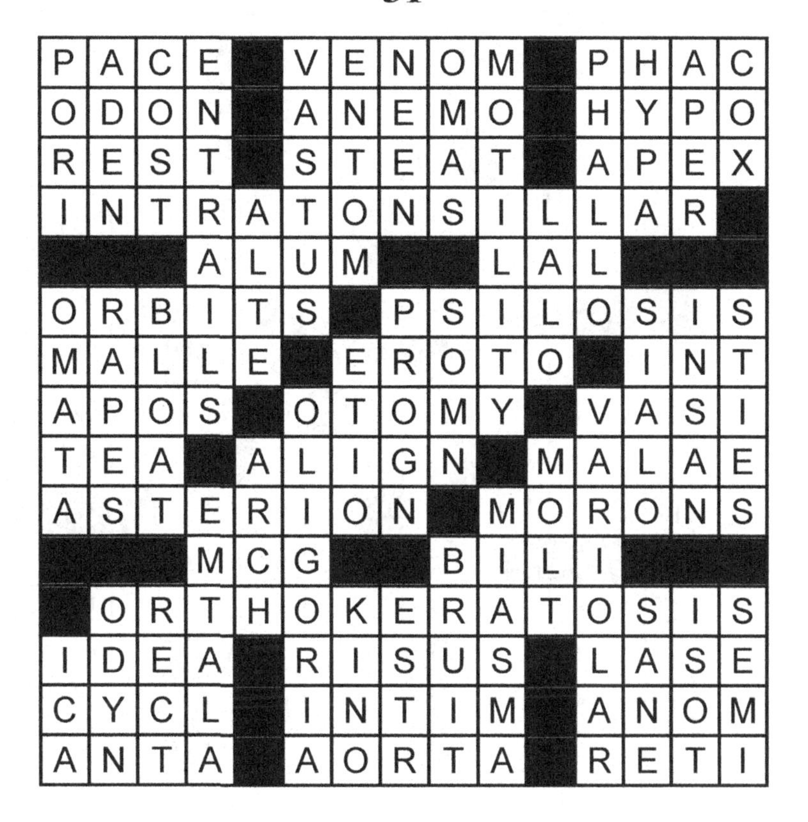
PACE VENOM PHAC
ODON ANEMO HYPO
REST STEAT APEX
INTRATONSILLAR
ALUM LAL
ORBITS PSILOSIS
MALLE EROTO INT
APOS OTOMY VASI
TEA ALIGN MALAE
ASTERION MORONS
MCG BILI
ORTHOKERATOSIS
IDEA RISUS LASE
CYCL INTIM ANOM
ANTA AORTA RETI

32

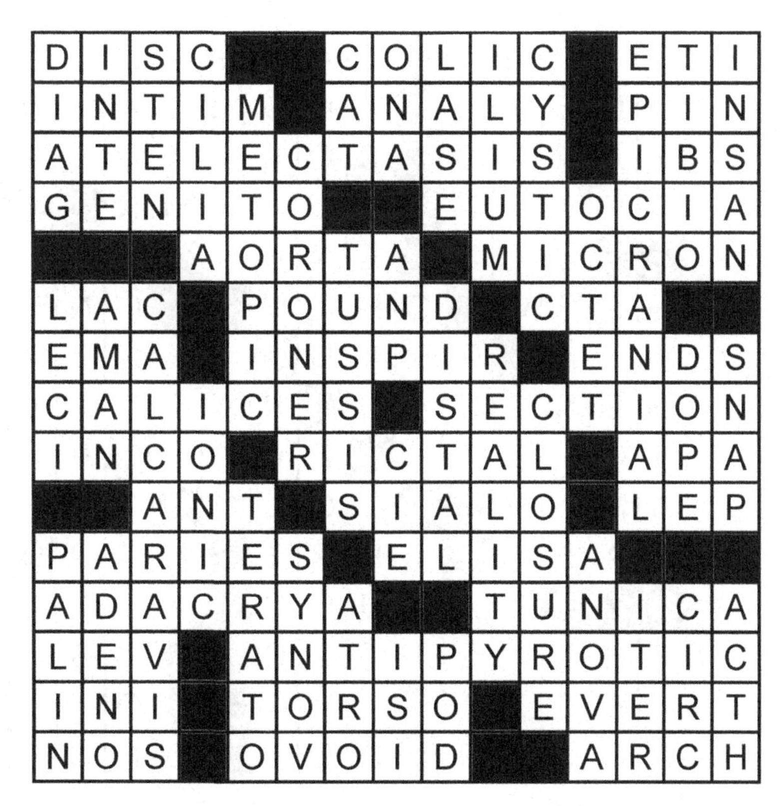
DISC COLIC ETI
INTIM ANALY PIN
ATELECTASIS IBS
GENITO EUTOCIA
AORTA MICRON
LAC POUND CTA
EMA INSPIR ENDS
CALICES SECTION
INCO RICTAL APA
ANT SIALO LEP
PARIES ELISA
ADACRYA TUNICA
LEV ANTIPYROTIC
INI TORSO EVERT
NOS OVOID ARCH

33

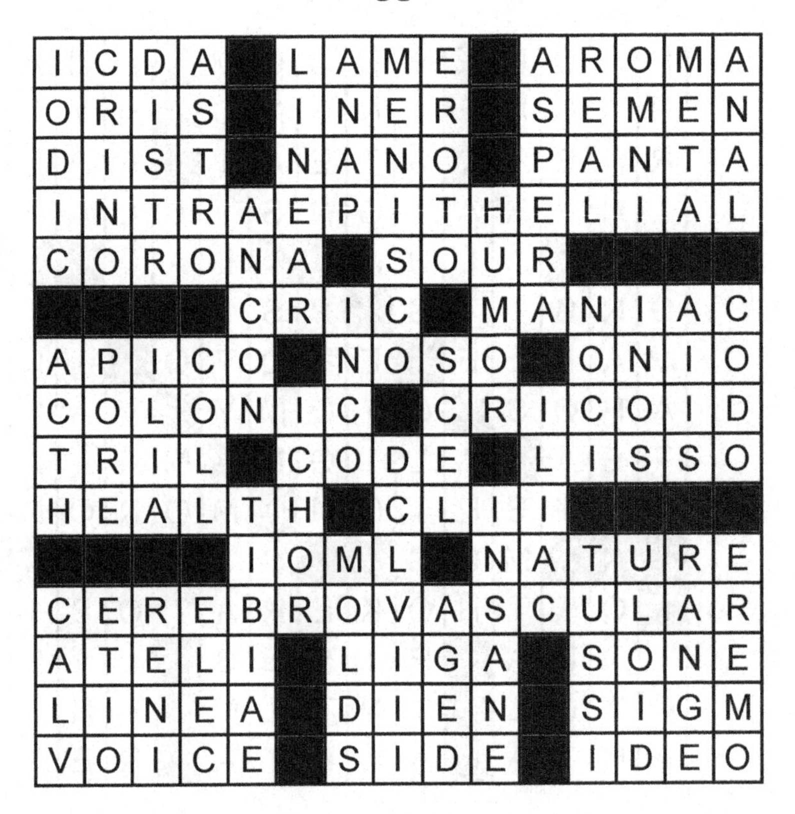

I	C	D	A	■	L	A	M	E	■	A	R	O	M	A
O	R	I	S	■	I	N	E	R	■	S	E	M	E	N
D	I	S	T	■	N	A	N	O	■	P	A	N	T	A
I	N	T	R	A	E	P	I	T	H	E	L	I	A	L
C	O	R	O	N	A	■	S	O	U	R	■	■	■	■
■	■	■	■	C	R	I	C	■	M	A	N	I	A	C
A	P	I	C	O	■	N	O	S	O	■	O	N	I	O
C	O	L	O	N	I	C	■	C	R	I	C	O	I	D
T	R	I	L	■	C	O	D	E	■	L	I	S	S	O
H	E	A	L	T	H	■	C	L	I	I	■	■	■	■
■	■	■	■	I	O	M	L	■	N	A	T	U	R	E
C	E	R	E	B	R	O	V	A	S	C	U	L	A	R
A	T	E	L	I	■	L	I	G	A	■	S	O	N	E
L	I	N	E	A	■	D	I	E	N	■	S	I	G	M
V	O	I	C	E	■	S	I	D	E	■	I	D	E	O

34

R	A	P	H	E	■	V	A	C	■	N	O	T	A	L
O	N	E	I	R	■	I	N	O	■	O	P	I	N	E
T	A	R	S	O	■	S	C	L	E	R	I	T	I	S
S	P	I	T	S	■	C	O	L	U	M	N	■	■	■
■	■	C	I	E	■	E	N	U	R	■	I	A	H	S
M	E	R	O	■	G	R	A	M	■	■	O	N	E	I
A	L	A	■	G	R	A	D	■	P	E	N	T	A	D
M	E	N	S	U	A	L	■	P	A	S	S	I	V	E
M	O	I	E	T	Y	■	F	E	R	R	■	P	E	R
A	M	A	N	■	■	C	O	L	O	■	M	Y	S	O
L	A	L	I	■	I	R	R	I	■	N	O	R	■	■
■	■	■	L	A	N	U	G	O	■	A	T	E	L	I
C	H	E	I	L	I	T	I	S	■	R	I	S	U	S
L	E	C	T	A	■	C	V	I	■	C	O	I	T	O
A	R	G	Y	R	■	H	E	S	■	O	N	S	E	T

35

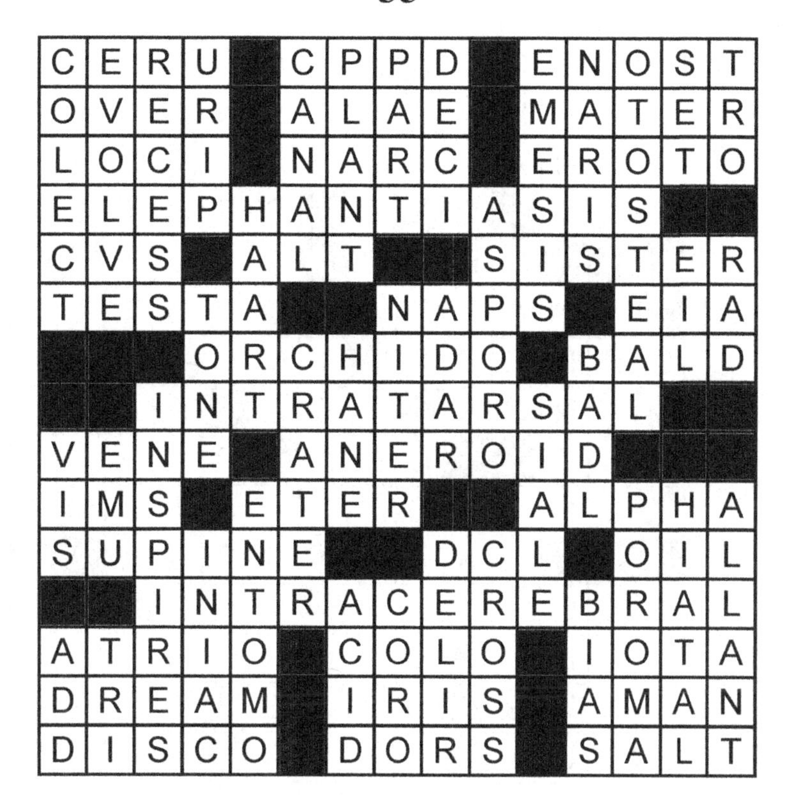

36

P	A	T	H	O		S	N	A	P		H	E	M	E
O	B	E	Y	S		P	O	N	S		O	L	I	G
D	I	A	S	T		O	C	T	I		M	I	T	E
	O	S	T	E	O	D	I	A	S	T	A	S	I	S
			E	O	S	O				E	L	A	S	T
L	E	A	R	N	S		L	A	L	I	O			
I	R	R	I			I	O	N	I	C		D	S	M
N	O	T	A	N	E	N	C	E	P	H	A	L	I	A
I	S	I		I	N	I	A	C			B	I	D	S
			S	T	O	O	L		P	A	R	I	E	S
M	I	S	C	E				H	E	P	A			
E	N	T	E	R	O	S	T	E	N	O	S	I	S	
S	T	E	N		R	E	A	L		D	I	C	O	M
A	O	R	T		C	L	I	I		I	O	D	I	C
D	E	N	S		H	A	L	O		A	N	A	L	G

37

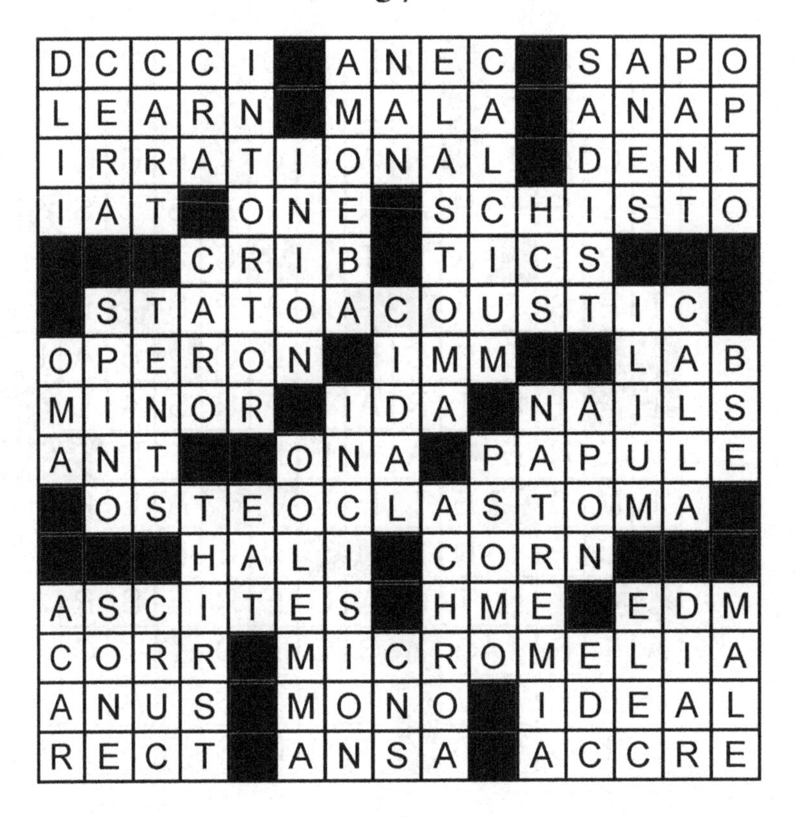
DCCCI ANEC SAPO
LEARN MALA ANAP
IRRATIONAL DENT
IAT ONE SCHISTO
CRIB TICS
STATOACOUSTIC
OPERON IMM LAB
MINOR IDA NAILS
ANT ONA PAPULE
OSTEOCLASTOMA
HALI CORN
ASCITES HME EDM
CORR MICROMELIA
ANUS MONO IDEAL
RECT ANSA ACCRE

38

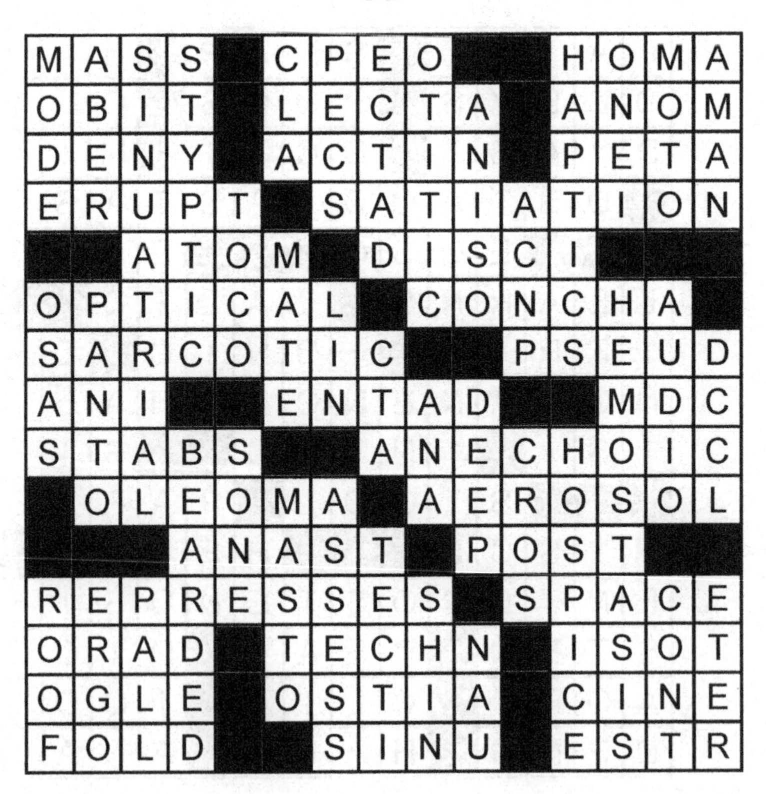
MASS CPEO HOMA
OBIT LECTA ANOM
DENY ACTIN PETA
ERUPT SATIATION
ATOM DISCI
OPTICAL CONCHA
SARCOTIC PSEUD
ANI ENTAD MDC
STABS ANECHOIC
OLEOMA AEROSOL
ANAST POST
REPRESSES SPACE
ORAD TECHN ISOT
OGLE OSTIA CINE
FOLD SINU ESTR

39

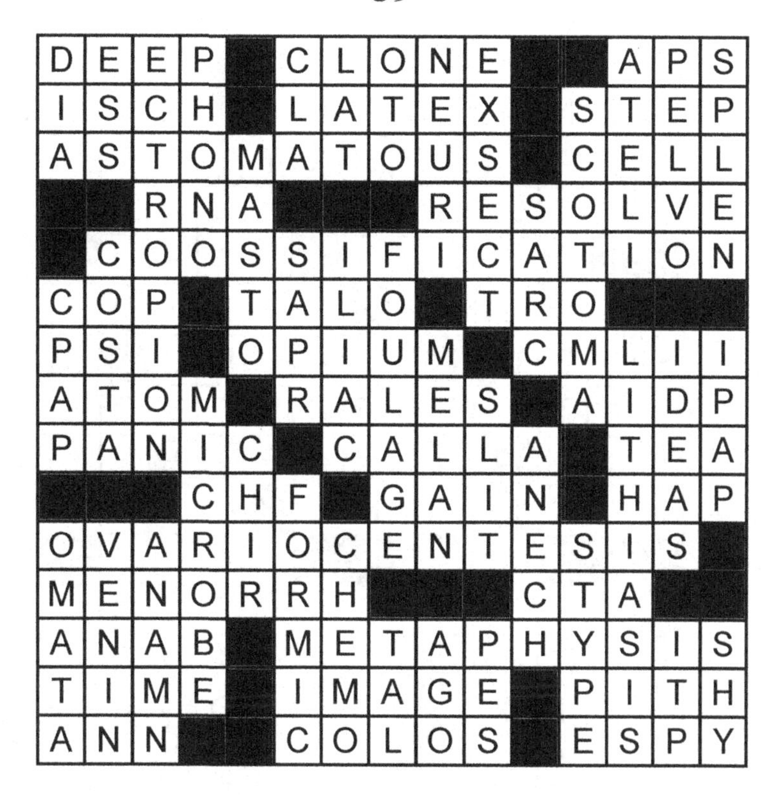

D	E	E	P		C	L	O	N	E			A	P	S
I	S	C	H		L	A	T	E	X		S	T	E	P
A	S	T	O	M	A	T	O	U	S		C	E	L	L
		R	N	A				R	E	S	O	L	V	E
	C	O	O	S	S	I	F	I	C	A	T	I	O	N
C	O	P		T	A	L	O		T	R	O			
P	S	I		O	P	I	U	M		C	M	L	I	I
A	T	O	M		R	A	L	E	S		A	I	D	P
P	A	N	I	C		C	A	L	L	A		T	E	A
			C	H	F		G	A	I	N		H	A	P
O	V	A	R	I	O	C	E	N	T	E	S	I	S	
M	E	N	O	R	R	H				C	T	A		
A	N	A	B		M	E	T	A	P	H	Y	S	I	S
T	I	M	E		I	M	A	G	E		P	I	T	H
A	N	N			C	O	L	O	S		E	S	P	Y

40

O	M	A	S		S	T	U	N	S		I	M	P	E
M	E	G	A		P	E	N	I	A		N	E	O	N
P	L	A	N		A	L	I	G	N		I	R	I	D
H	E	M	I	G	N	A	T	H	I	A		O	S	A
A	N	I	O	N			S	T	E	N		G	O	N
L	A	C		A	M	L			S	T	R	O	N	G
			S	T	R	U	M	I			A	N	S	I
		A	P	H	A	S	I	O	L	O	G	Y		
T	O	C	O			I	O	D	I	N	E			
R	O	T	T	E	D			O	M	S		L	E	S
I	P	I		T	E	L	O			E	R	U	C	T
C	L	V		I	N	A	P	P	E	T	E	N	C	E
H	A	I	R		I	N	T	I	M		A	U	R	A
I	S	T	H		A	C	I	N	I		C	L	I	T
A	M	Y	O		L	E	C	T	A		T	E	N	O

41

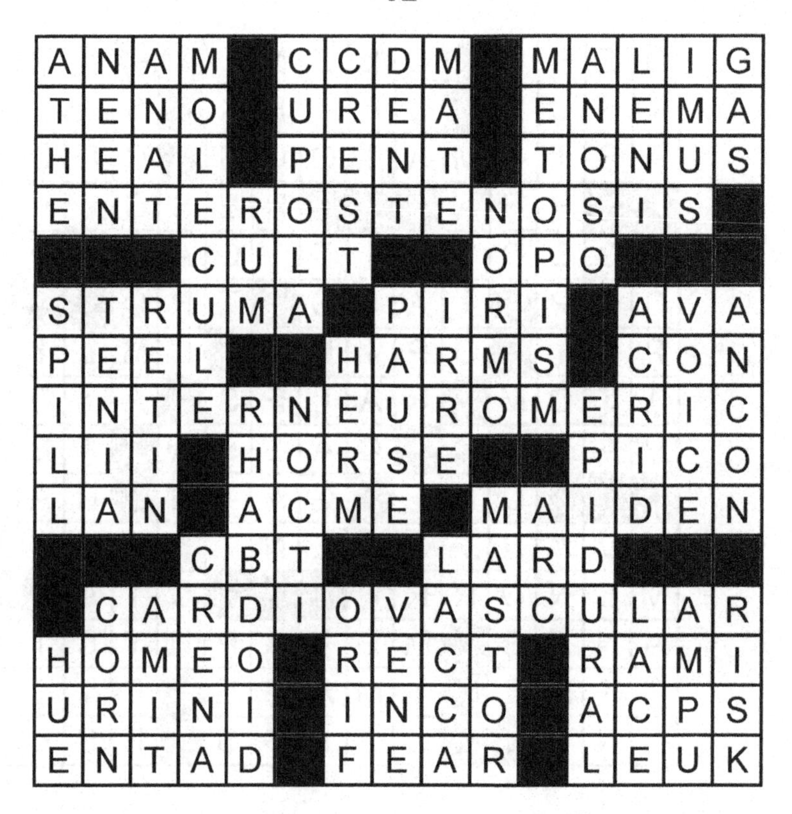
ANAM CCDM MALIG
TENO UREA ENEMA
HEAL PENT TONUS
ENTEROSTENOSIS
CULT OPO
STRUMA PIRI AVA
PEEL HARMS CON
INTERNEUROMERIC
LII HORSE PICO
LAN ACME MAIDEN
CBT LARD
CARDIOVASCULAR
HOMEO RECT RAMI
URINI INCO ACPS
ENTAD FEAR LEUK

42

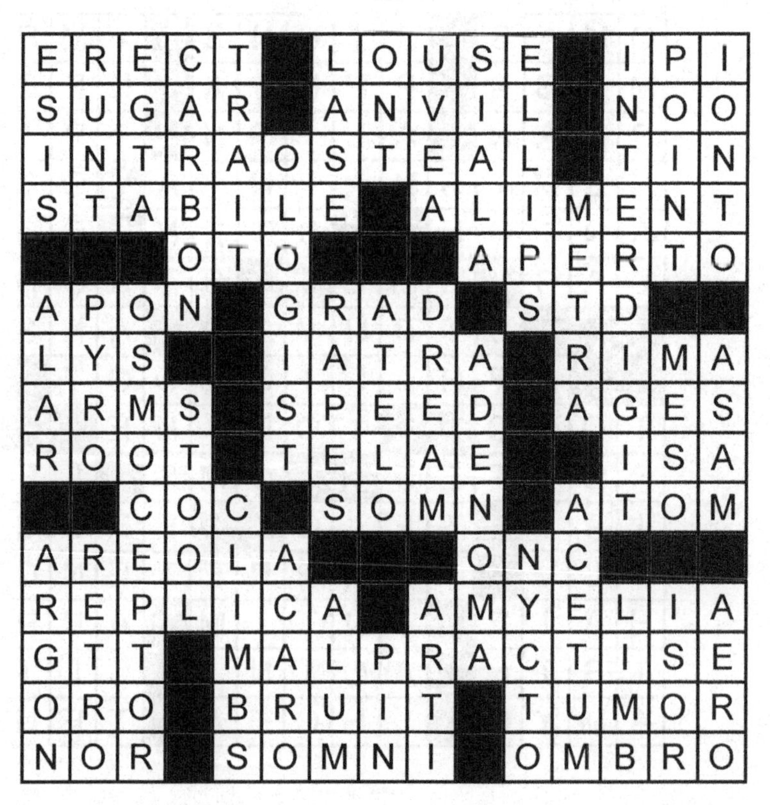
ERECT LOUSE IPI
SUGAR ANVIL NOO
INTRAOSTEAL TIN
STABILE ALIMENT
OTO APERTO
APON GRAD STD
LYS IATRA RIMA
ARMS SPEED AGES
ROOT TELAE ISA
COC SOMN ATOM
AREOLA ONC
REPLICA AMYELIA
GTT MALPRACTISE
ORO BRUIT TUMOR
NOR SOMNI OMBRO

43

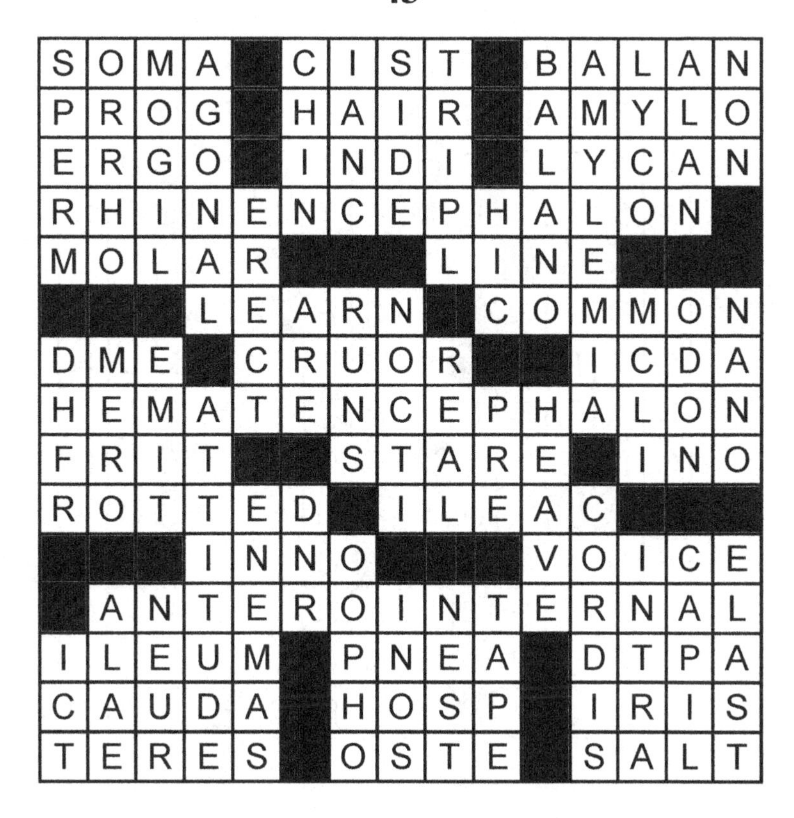

S	O	M	A		C	I	S	T		B	A	L	A	N
P	R	O	G		H	A	I	R		A	M	Y	L	O
E	R	G	O		I	N	D	I		L	Y	C	A	N
R	H	I	N	E	N	C	E	P	H	A	L	O	N	
M	O	L	A	R				L	I	N	E			
			L	E	A	R	N		C	O	M	M	O	N
D	M	E		C	R	U	O	R			I	C	D	A
H	E	M	A	T	E	N	C	E	P	H	A	L	O	N
F	R	I	T			S	T	A	R	E		I	N	O
R	O	T	T	E	D		I	L	E	A	C			
			I	N	N	O				V	O	I	C	E
	A	N	T	E	R	O	I	N	T	E	R	N	A	L
I	L	E	U	M		P	N	E	A		D	T	P	A
C	A	U	D	A		H	O	S	P		I	R	I	S
T	E	R	E	S		O	S	T	E		S	A	L	T

44

M	C	V	I		F	I	R	S	T		C	I	R	C
O	L	E	N		A	R	A	C	H		A	D	E	N
T	I	N	T		N	I	T	E	R		P	E	P	S
I	N	T	R	A	A	D	E	N	O	I	D	A	L	
V	I	R	A	L				E	B	V		T	A	P
E	C	O		A	L	U	M		S	U	P	I	N	E
			C	R	A	V	A	T			R	O	T	S
		E	M	A	C	U	L	A	T	I	O	N		
O	M	N	I			L	I	P	I	D	S			
M	O	T	I	L	E		G	E	N	E		A	H	A
A	N	O		I	T	P				A	S	T	E	R
	O	P	H	T	H	A	L	M	O	S	C	O	P	Y
E	C	T	O		I	N	I	A	D		A	N	A	T
I	L	I	O		C	O	C	C	Y		B	I	T	E
N	E	C	K		S	T	E	R	N		S	C	A	N

45

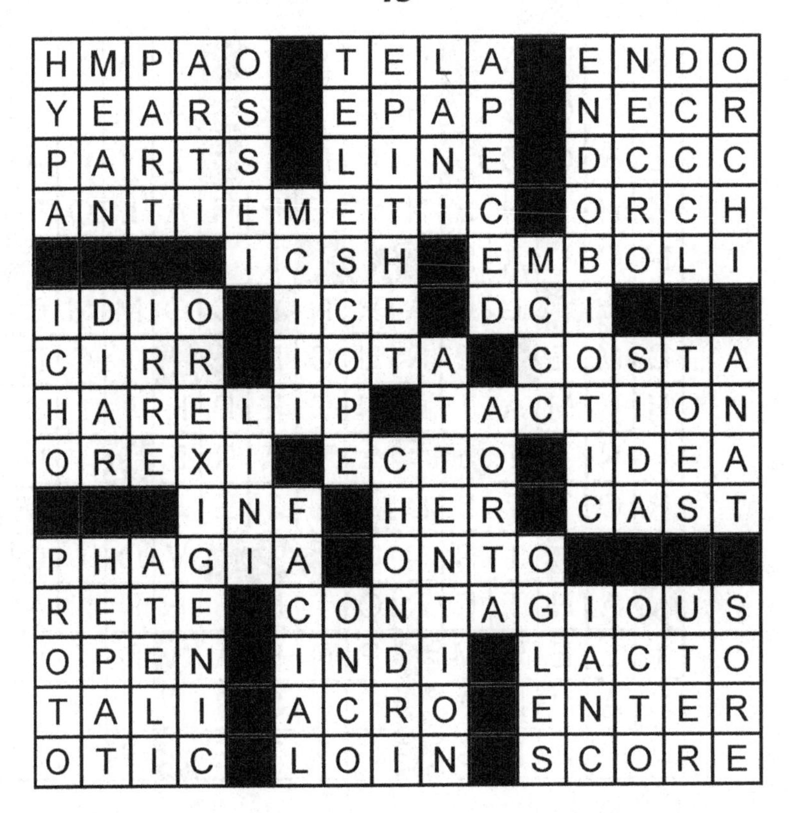
HMPAO TELA ENDO
YEARS EPAP NECR
PARTS LINE DCCC
ANTIEMETIC ORCH
ICSH EMBOLI
IDIO ICE DCI
CIRR IOTA COSTA
HARELIP TACTION
OREXI ECTO IDEA
INF HER CAST
PHAGIA ONTO
RETE CONTAGIOUS
OPEN INDI LACTO
TALI ACRO ENTER
OTIC LOIN SCORE

46

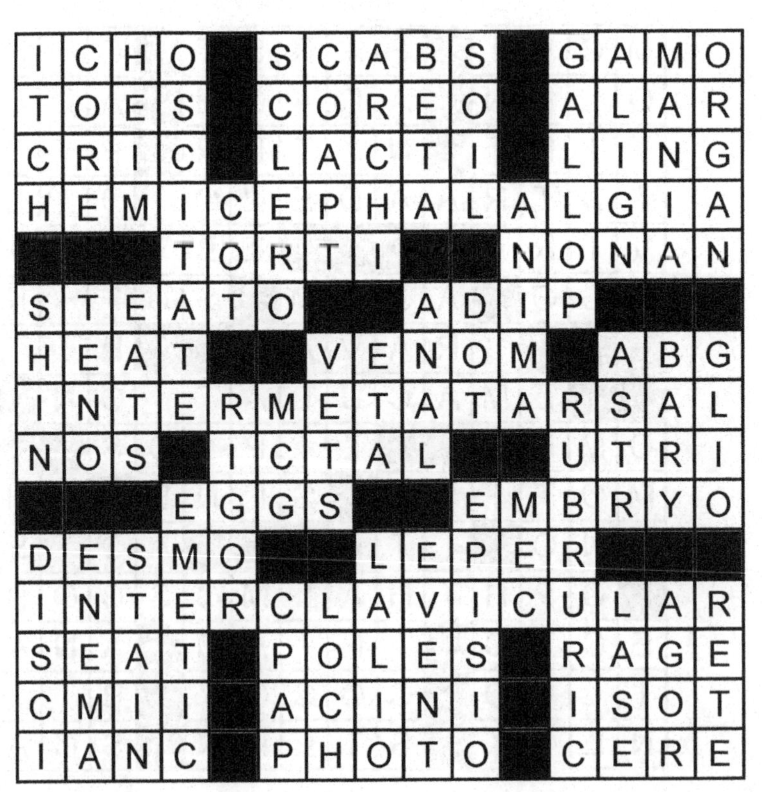
ICHO SCABS GAMO
TOES COREO ALAR
CRIC LACTI LING
HEMICEPHALALGIA
TORTI NONAN
STEATO ADIP
HEAT VENOM ABG
INTERMETATARSAL
NOS ICTAL UTRI
EGGS EMBRYO
DESMO LEPER
INTERCLAVICULAR
SEAT POLES RAGE
CMII ACINI ISOT
IANC PHOTO CERE

47

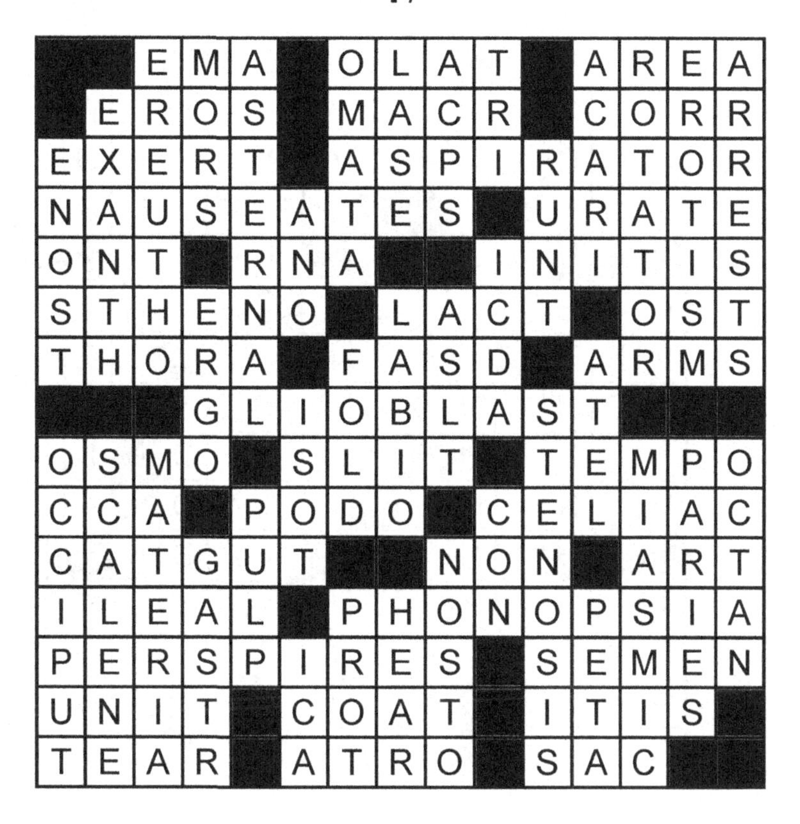

48

A	N	T	U		S	O	M	A		I	S	C	H	I
N	E	E	N		O	V	E	R		M	E	L	A	N
T	O	N	E		M	A	L	T		M	L	I	I	I
I	N	T	R	A	A	R	T	I	C	U	L	A	R	
			U	R	T	I			O	N	A			
K	L	E	P	T	O		C	I	L	I		M	E	L
N	I	N	T	H		P	O	R	E		M	O	X	A
I	N	T	E	R	N	E	U	R	O	M	E	R	I	C
F	E	E	D		A	N	G	I		E	N	O	S	T
E	A	R		O	R	T	H		O	D	O	N	T	O
			D	C	C			S	P	I	R			
	E	M	E	T	O	C	A	T	H	A	R	T	I	C
A	T	E	L	O		I	N	E	R		H	E	A	L
T	E	S	T	S		D	E	N	Y		E	N	D	O
E	R	O	S	E		E	C	T	O		A	S	L	T

49

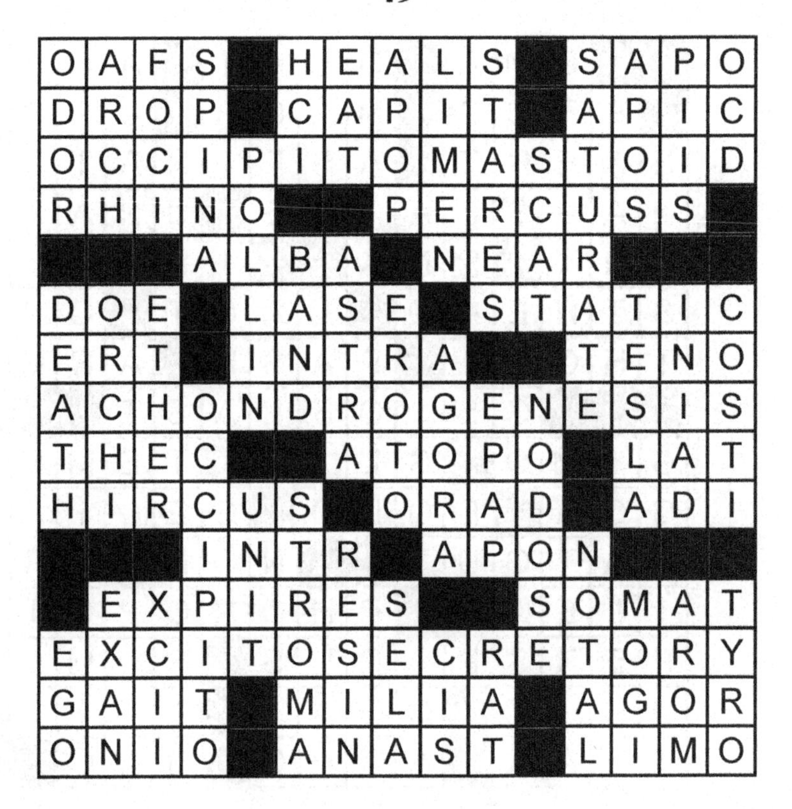

50

O	R	I	S		S	A	P	O		P	H	A	G	O
V	E	N	O		C	M	H	C		H	Y	P	O	G
I	N	T	R	A	M	Y	O	C	A	R	D	I	A	L
N	A	R	E	S			T	U	B	E	R	C	L	E
E	L	A	S	T	I	N		L	I	N				
					M	A	S	T	O		A	P	O	S
I	S	C	H	E	M	I	C			S	C	A	L	E
A	U	R	I	C	U	L	O	C	R	A	N	I	A	L
D	R	O	P	S			P	L	A	C	E	N	T	A
L	A	S	S		W	H	O	O	P					
				M	I	O		T	E	R	T	I	A	N
C	E	P	H	A	L	A	D			U	R	A	N	O
A	C	H	O	N	D	R	O	G	E	N	E	S	I	S
S	T	O	R	I		S	T	E	N		M	I	M	E
T	O	N	I	A		E	E	N	T		O	S	A	S

Made in the USA
Coppell, TX
17 April 2022